'Catherine G. Lucas's *Coping with a Mer*
healing points the way towards understan_
as part of the human search for meaning and inner truth. As such, the _
ferer need not adopt the hopelessness of psychiatry's brain illness model.
Her advice for those seeking help makes this book a must-read.'

Daniel Dorman, MD, Assistant Clinical Professor of Psychiatry
UCLA School of Medicine, and author of *Dante's Cure:*
A journey out of madness

'Can a mental health crisis ever be a blessing in disguise? In this handbook
for healing, Catherine G. Lucas offers advice that's practical, holistic and
gently optimistic, grown out of her own personal experience and resonating
strongly with the work I do being alongside some of the world's most sensitive and spiritual people; mental-health service users. For anyone who is
willing to make the choice to take responsibility for their own recovery, this
book will be both unique and invaluable, describing a wide variety of transformative ways to harness the potential for light even in the darkest of places.'

Mirabai Swingler, Spiritual Care Leader
North East London NHS Foundation Trust (NELFT)
and founder of the Only Us campaign

'Catherine G. Lucas provides a very comprehensive set of complementary
alternatives to the biomedical model for someone experiencing a mental
health crisis. As a person with "lived experience", she speaks with authority
when she says you need to make sure the person you choose to support
and guide you believes you can get better. This is a must-read for people
experiencing a mental health crisis or for those looking for an effective way
to support them.'

Phil Borges, Director, *CrazyWise*

'Catherine brings a long overdue, compassionate and thoughtful challenge
to the standard view that so-called mental illness is simply a pathology,
with the only recourse being a lifetime of medication and psychiatry. It's a
call to recognize the spiritual component of apparent "psychosis", seeing
it rather as an opportunity for soul-level healing: a massive and deep reorganization of the psyche necessary for radical transformation. It builds on
the insights in her previous book, and offers practical and achievable advice
on how to live well and heal from a psychological crisis.'

Richard Drake, Spiritual Emergence Service (Canada)
and author of *Nirvana by Installments*

Coping with a Mental Health Crisis

Catherine G. Lucas is an accredited mindfulness trainer, working both face to face and online. She has been training groups since 2007, including NHS therapists, as well as soldiers returning from Iraq and Afghanistan, for the Ministry of Defence. Catherine is also author of *In Case of Spiritual Emergency* and founder of the Spiritual Crisis Network, a UK charity. Catherine is a respected international speaker on psychospiritual crisis and active in building international collaboration in the field.

Overcoming Common Problems Series

Selected titles

A full list of titles is available from Sheldon Press,
36 Causton Street, London SW1P 4ST and on our website at
www.sheldonpress.co.uk

Breast Cancer: Your treatment choices
Dr Terry Priestman

Chronic Fatigue Syndrome: What you need to know about CFS/ME
Dr Megan A. Arroll

Cider Vinegar
Margaret Hills

Coeliac Disease: What you need to know
Alex Gazzola

Coping Successfully with Hiatus Hernia
Dr Tom Smith

Coping with Difficult Families
Dr Jane McGregor and Tim McGregor

Coping with Epilepsy
Dr Pamela Crawford and Fiona Marshall

Coping with Memory Problems
Dr Sallie Baxendale

Coping with the Psychological Effects of Illness
Dr Fran Smith, Dr Carina Eriksen
and Professor Robert Bor

Coping with Schizophrenia
Professor Kevin Gournay and Debbie Robson

Coping with Thyroid Disease
Mark Greener

Depressive Illness: The curse of the strong
Dr Tim Cantopher

Dr Dawn's Guide to Brain Health
Dr Dawn Harper

Dr Dawn's Guide to Heart Health
Dr Dawn Harper

Dr Dawn's Guide to Weight and Diabetes
Dr Dawn Harper

Dr Dawn's Guide to Women's Health
Dr Dawn Harper

The Empathy Trap: Understanding antisocial personalities
Dr Jane McGregor and Tim McGregor

The Fibromyalgia Healing Diet
Christine Craggs-Hinton

Fibromyalgia: Your treatment guide
Christine Craggs-Hinton

Helping Elderly Relatives
Jill Eckersley

The Holistic Health Handbook
Mark Greener

How to Stop Worrying
Dr Frank Tallis

Invisible Illness: Coping with misunderstood conditions
Dr Megan A. Arroll and Professor
Christine P. Dancey

Living with the Challenges of Dementia: A guide for family and friends
Patrick McCurry

Living with Complicated Grief
Professor Craig A. White

Living with Fibromyalgia
Christine Craggs-Hinton

Living with Hearing Loss
Dr Don McFerran, Lucy Handscomb
and Dr Cherilee Rutherford

Overcoming Fear with Mindfulness
Deborah Ward

Overcoming Low Self-esteem with Mindfulness
Deborah Ward

Overcoming Stress
Professor Robert Bor, Dr Carina Eriksen
and Dr Sara Chaudry

Overcoming Worry and Anxiety
Dr Jerry Kennard

Physical Intelligence: How to take charge of your weight
Dr Tom Smith

Post-Traumatic Stress Disorder: Recovery after accident and disaster
Professor Kevin Gournay

The Self-Esteem Journal
Alison Waines

The Stroke Survival Guide
Mark Greener

Ten Steps to Positive Living
Dr Windy Dryden

Treating Arthritis: The drug-free way
Margaret Hills and Christine Horner

Understanding High Blood Pressure
Dr Shahid Aziz and Dr Zara Aziz

Understanding Yourself and Others: Practical ideas from the world of coaching
Bob Thomson

When Someone You Love Has Depression: A handbook for family and friends
Barbara Baker

Overcoming Common Problems

Coping with a Mental Health Crisis

Seven steps to healing

CATHERINE G. LUCAS

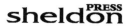
sheldon PRESS

First published in Great Britain in 2015

Sheldon Press
36 Causton Street
London SW1P 4ST
www.sheldonpress.co.uk

The author and publisher have made every effort to ensure that the
external website and email addresses included in this book are correct and
up to date at the time of going to press. The author and publisher are not
responsible for the content, quality or continuing accessibility of the sites.

British Library Cataloguing-in-Publication Data
A catalogue record for this book is available from the British Library

ISBN 978–1–84709–307–3
eBook ISBN 978–1–84709–308–0

Typeset by Fakenham Prepress Solutions, Fakenham, Norfolk NR21 8NN
First printed in Great Britain by Ashford Colour Press
Subsequently digitally reprinted in Great Britain

eBook by Fakenham Prepress Solutions, Fakenham, Norfolk NR21 8NN

Produced on paper from sustainable forests

For you

I've written this book because I believe in you.
I believe in your ability to heal and grow.
I believe in your ability to wake up, to become self-aware,
to move towards love and away from fear.
I believe in your ability to take ownership of your journey
towards wholeness.
I believe in your courage, determination and perseverance,
all of which you will need to succeed on this journey.
Above all, I believe you. I believe your experience.
I believe it has a deeper meaning, a soulful meaning.
I honour that and I honour you.

Contents

Foreword

Catherine G. Lucas has written a very important book and has given us a precious gift. Since the beginning of biological psychiatry in the late 1950s through the 'Decade of the Brain' in the 1990s to now, the mind, body and spirit connection as it relates to extreme mental states has been sorely missing. In many ways it has been relegated to the realms of irrelevancy by mainstream psychiatry.

The focus on brain pathology and chemical imbalances has led to a mental health paradigm of care that tends to negate the deeper meaning and purpose of an individual's lived experience. In her book, which is both comprehensive and informative, Catherine gives compelling evidence through personal stories, including her own. These show that going through a serious mental health challenge can be a catalyst for change, an opportunity for healing and growth, rather than a lifetime sentence of symptom management where downward spirals are considered the norm, as is the control of such downward spirals with potent psychoactive medication.

Working in the mental health field for 32 years as a psychiatric nurse, trainer and supervisor, I have seen how a reductionist approach which focuses more on a diagnostic label has contributed to the despair and hopelessness felt by so many people going through extreme state. A person is much more than a collection of symptoms. Healing requires an integrated whole-person approach, one in which not only the person but also that person's unique lived experience is valued.

Catherine gives examples of different therapeutic approaches and modalities which honour the role of soul or spirit in a mental health crisis. I have come to realize at a most profound level that what is much thought of (falsely so) as pathology and an illness has its roots in wounds of the soul. It is because of the significance those wounds have on the one experiencing them, which largely goes unaddressed, that I resonate so much with Catherine's book.

At 18, I felt my mind was leaving me. Intrusive voices were telling me to harm myself and those I loved. Living with a father who was mentally and emotionally abusive took its toll. At school I was teased and made fun of, which made me feel worse and even more alone. I was falling down a deep, dark hole with no end in sight to the pain and suffering.

It was the late 1960s and I was diagnosed with what my parents were told was an incurable mental disorder. For the next year and a half I was hospitalized twice and put on heavy doses of psychotropic medication with symptom suppression as the primary focus. As my despair worsened, so did the debilitating side effects of the medications I was on.

It was during my third and last hospitalization, lasting over three years, that things began to change. The psychiatrist assigned to me, also a trained psychotherapist, treated me differently. He showed interest in me and believed in my ability to heal. Instead of prescribing medication, he listened. Although I was silent during most of the first year of therapy and rarely talked, he never gave up on me. My feelings and experiences were validated. Later, when I asked him why he always stayed the entire 55 minutes of our therapy sessions when I didn't appear to be responding, he told me that he felt there was meaning in my silence. During the remainder of my hospitalization, including four years of therapy afterwards with the same therapist, I embarked on a journey of growth and self-discovery that I continue to benefit from to this very day. The psychospiritual crisis I had experienced opened me up to life.

It was sheer culture shock when I began working as a psychiatric nurse in the late 1970s. People going through severe mental emotional distress and given labels such as 'schizophrenia', as I had once been given, were heavily medicated, many times against their will. Talking therapies were not available to those with such labels because the psychiatric community deemed that people with certain diagnoses would not benefit from them. Psychosocial therapies were limited.

More times than not, medications were given as punishment and a means of maintaining control by the nursing staff rather than as a valid therapeutic intervention. On numerous occasions I was told that I spent too much time with 'patients', that their delusions had no meaning and their behaviours would only intensify if I gave them too much attention. Early on I had to ask myself: did I really want to continue working as a psychiatric nurse in a healthcare field where the environment so disregarded and undervalued a person's humanity?

My answer came when I remembered the difference that one person made in my life by just being there, engendering hope and a will to live, not merely to survive, through compassionate empathetic care.

Within the last 15 years there has been a slow shift in the mental health field towards a paradigm of care that is starting to recognize the value of a whole-person approach as it relates to people going through serious mental health challenges. A large part of that shift can be credited to the recovery model of care, with a focus on a person's strengths rather than symptoms. People's lived experience and how they relate to that experience is being included in treatment planning and considered a vital part of those strengths. Psychosocial therapies are gaining prominence. Long-term maintenance on psychiatric drugs is being scrutinized as more evidence and research is revealing that the duration of antipsychotic treatment leads to significant increases in cardiometabolic risk factors, risk factors which contribute to higher mortality and morbidity rates.

Because of these changes, and especially in the context of the broader therapeutic community, this book is extremely significant and timely. There are many paths to healing and wellness that are transformative and soul enriching, as Catherine illustrates so eloquently: paths which emphasize resiliency and the innate striving within us all not just to survive a serious psychological crisis, but to thrive on a mental, emotional and spiritual level from having gone through one.

How people come to view their experience, whether it be as life-affirming or life-threatening, has much to do with the attitudes of the professionals working with people in crisis and their belief in those people's ability to heal. Catherine addresses these issues and much more, providing options, strategies and resources to help on the journey. The transpersonal nature and deeper meaning of severe psychic distress and the role it plays in developing a sense of purpose in life; the importance of a supportive nurturing environment, including counsellor or therapist; and the therapeutic value of a balanced approach, are all intricately woven into the fabric of this book.

Finally, *Coping with a Mental Crisis: Seven steps to healing* inspires hope and empowerment. At the same time, it draws our attention to how important it is for the mental health community to continue its growing trend towards a vision of care that embraces a more holistic path, one in which the person is valued as the main influencer of his or her own care.

Catherine Penney, RN, California

Catherine Penney is featured in Dante's Cure: A journey out of madness *by Dr Daniel Dorman.*

Acknowledgements

I'd like to thank Fiona, at Sheldon Press, for her vision in commissioning this book and for giving me the opportunity to contribute to the rising swell of change within mental health. Thank you for helping to bring this book to those who need it. As an editor, you have a wonderful skill of naturally and effortlessly balancing support with hands-off trust.

Heartfelt thanks go to all those who have shared their experiences for the benefit of others, especially Hamilton, Jane and Ursula, as well as Marie and Mary. Thank you for your act of service. I am also deeply honoured and grateful to Cathy Penney for writing the Foreword. Thank you for such a generous gift, Cathy. You are a truly inspiring woman!

When I met my husband, I didn't realize just how important his background in journalism would turn out to be. It has meant that his unfailing, total and utter support of me and the book has been not simply emotional but also extremely practical and real. Thank you, Swithin, for your professional, discerning judgement on all things writerly. Thank you for your infectious love of the creative life.

Finally, I would like to thank Dr Andrew Weil for his book *Spontaneous Healing*, which I read many moons ago. His chapter on the seven strategies of successful patients made a deep impression on me and was the inspiration for my 'Seven steps to healing'.

Note to the reader

Please take good care of yourself while reading this book. Be sure to seek medical care and professional mental health advice when you need it. This book is not intended to replace that or to be used as a handbook for treatment.

The names of those who have generously shared their personal experience have been changed.

All details of books and articles discussed can be found in the 'Further reading' or 'References' sections, and all websites are listed in 'Useful addresses', all at the end of the book.

COPING WITH A MENTAL HEALTH CRISIS

The life you want to live

This is a book about healing and growth. It is about taking charge of your life, creating the healing you want to see, the life you want to live. It is based on my healing journey and that of others, those of us who have experience in how to heal and grow. One of these is Cathy Penney. I invited this inspiring woman to write the Foreword because she is the living embodiment of this book's message: you can heal. *Coping with a Mental Health Crisis* is also based on my professional expertise of supporting others on their healing journeys through the mindfulness training and mentoring I offer.

Who is this book for?

This book is for you if:

- you have been through a mental health crisis;
- you are looking for ways to make sense of what you have been through;
- you've had a mental health crisis and want to use it as an opportunity for healing and growth, to help make sure it doesn't happen again;
- you are willing to take responsibility for moving successfully through this challenging time in your life, if you are willing to actively engage with the 'Seven steps to healing';
- following a mental health crisis, you have discovered a newfound interest in spirituality because of what you've been through;
- a loved one, friend or colleague has been through a mental health crisis and you want to support that person as effectively as possible;
- you work in the field of mental health or you work as a practitioner in any health-related field and come across patients or clients experiencing mental distress;
- as a practitioner, you are looking for a more holistic approach to mental health and feel that reducing everything to chemical imbalance in the brain is not creating the wellbeing you hope to see in your patients and clients;
- as a practitioner, you are interested in an integrative approach, combining complimentary and new science healing modalities with the best of mainstream care;
- as a member of the broader public, you care about how we treat those going through mental health crisis.

Why is this book needed?

- Because if you're recovering from a mental health crisis you need to be well informed. You need to know that you have options, that you can create a package of integrative mental health care bringing together the very best of mainstream and complimentary approaches, individually tailored to your needs.
- Because 'psychiatry' comes from the ancient Greek meaning 'healing of the soul' and this book puts the soul back into mental health.
- Because the world is rapidly changing, as is mental health care. Quantum physics has now proved that we are all connected through one single energetic field, that we are all part of one interconnected Whole. Many going through crisis touch into this and get a sense of it experientially. This spiritual aspect of a mental health crisis needs honouring because it holds the key to healing.
- Because, as the world and mental health rapidly develop, new therapeutic approaches are coming on board which successfully enable people to lead meaningful, fulfilling lives. To take just one example, Open Dialogue, which is based on hearing and considering what everyone involved in the crisis, including family members, feel and want, has achieved remarkable results in its native Finland.
- Because many directly experience an aspect of spirituality within their crisis. This book helps readers to make sense of that.
- Because psychiatry is in crisis. The work of authors such as Robert Whitaker in the USA and James Davies in the UK has brought our attention to the shortfalls in orthodox care, the focus on managing symptoms rather than assisting real healing, the dangers of long-term use of psychiatric drugs and the damage caused by the profit motive of the pharmaceutical industry. The result is that many are now looking for deeper meaning and deeper healing, which this book supports.

My story

I come from a deeply wounded, dysfunctional family, a family that had no language for feelings. My father, whose own father died when he was two, was an alcoholic. To the outside world he was charming and charismatic; nobody knew he was hell to live with.

Eventually, I escaped to university. When I came home during the first Easter holidays I discovered that my family had disintegrated. My parents had split up and no-one had told me. That summer, my already fragile world collapsed. While my university friends worked and went off on trips abroad, I spent my summer holidays on an acute psychiatric ward.

It was a hugely traumatic time. I lost a year of my life. I spent most of it in bed struggling with the medication I was on, gradually tapering off, with regular appointments to see the psychiatrist I was under.

Afterwards, I got on with my life as best I could. I finished my degree, fell in love, went on to do a master's and got married. I tried not to ask too many questions, following the advice, albeit misguided, of the psychiatrist. But the niggling need to understand what had happened to me never totally went away.

My healing only really began ten years later when my husband and I split up. By then I had a full-time university post and was doing a PhD part-time. True to form, the crisis proved to be the catalyst I needed to embark on a journey of personal and spiritual growth. I decided to learn to meditate as a way of coping with the stress. That simple, small decision changed my entire life, my entire world. I signed up for a class and bought a 'teach yourself meditation' book, a short, introductory book which had a huge impact on me. It gave me sudden insight, when, in the last chapter, it described the states of consciousness which experienced meditators aspire to: feelings of unbounded love, bliss, peace. I instantly recognized such states from before I had ended up in hospital. I had known all along that something very important had happened to me, that there was more to my supposed breakdown than 'illness'.

During a routine follow-up appointment, I naively tried to explain these unitive states of consciousness to the psychiatrist, only to have my experiences dismissed. Fortunately, my meditation teacher recognized the importance of such states. He validated where the psychiatrist pathologized. When I subsequently found myself in crisis again, this was to prove to be a key factor: the distinction between those around me either pathologizing or validating what I was going through.

Along with my newfound sense of inner equilibrium, my meditation practice also gave me a sense of wanting to 'give something back'. I started doing voluntary work at the local psychiatric hospital for an independent advocacy project. There I learnt active listening skills, which encouraged me to take an introductory counselling course. I started to discover 'feelings'. I went on to do a six-month foundation in mindfulness-based psychotherapy at the Karuna Institute in Devon, followed by the first year of the professional training. In 2003, the intense healing work involved came to a head when I went on a group trip to Egypt. I found myself catapulted into psychospiritual crisis, or spiritual emergency as it is also known. I again experienced unitive states of consciousness, this time much more powerfully. I understood that I am so much more than this body called Catherine. I felt the bliss, the joy, the gratitude and peace that comes with this knowing. In that incredibly intense week, I experienced what felt like the entire suffering of humanity going back to the beginning of time. I also felt the love and compassion of the Virgin Mary flowing through me.

Under the strain of such emotional and psychological intensity my legs gave way and I couldn't walk. I ended up in a wheelchair for a few days and had to travel back to the UK like that. Although I lost touch with consensual reality for a day or two, the aftermath of this crisis was completely different from when I was at university.

The Karuna teaching staff and my therapist were totally supportive. They understood that this was a breakthrough, an opportunity for healing. The spiritual dimension was valued, not pathologized. Also, I had by then, thanks to the Karuna course, come across the material on transpersonal psychology and psychospiritual crisis which I'll be presenting here. This meant I had a spiritual context or frame of reference within which to make sense of what I had been through, something I most certainly did not have at the age of 20.

Instead of ending up in hospital, I took time off work to recover. A measure of how easily I regained my balance after such intensity is, I feel, the publication I co-created when I went back to work. *The Rainbow Journal*, by and for young people who self-injure, has helped thousands of youngsters since then and is still being published over ten years later.

In Egypt I saw for myself the power of my meditation and mindfulness practice to help me through. It helped me watch the antics of the mind. The terror my ego experienced as it dissolved led the mind to create distorted thinking. I was able to watch the relationship between fear and distorted thinking and gain enough distance, albeit not much, to help me cope. During another period of crisis in 2006, more intense than in 2003 and lasting a full month, I again saw the power of mindfulness in situations of acute crisis. As a result I decided to become a mindfulness trainer. I trained and was accredited the following year by Breathworks, who have trainers in 12 countries around the world. I've taught many groups since then, including NHS therapists and soldiers returning from Iraq and Afghanistan.

Along the way I set up the Spiritual Crisis Network (SCN), a UK charity whose aim is to raise awareness and understanding of psychospiritual crisis and to offer information and support to individuals, families and professionals. I also organized three residential conferences on spiritual emergency, with international speakers, at Hawkwood College near Stroud in Gloucestershire. I wrote *In Case of Spiritual Emergency*, which has been translated into Dutch by the publisher Ankh Hermes. All of this has come out of periods of crisis in 2003 and 2006 which were supported rather than pathologized. Admittedly, I had done a lot of personal therapy work to heal and strengthen an ego that suffered early damage in my family.

The growing and learning continues to this day but, at least for now, the most intense years of that journey are behind me. A testament to how far I've come is, I feel, the healthy and happy marriage I'm now blessed with. I had developed a penchant for entering into abusive and painful relationships – hardly surprising given my tortured relationship with my father. Thankfully those days are over.

Now, some 20 years after I unwittingly embarked on my healing path by enrolling on that meditation course, I can share with you an approach to mental health that I myself and so many others have benefited from so much.

A deeper understanding

To heal and grow we need to attend to the deeper needs of psyche and soul. So we take a holistic approach to our mental health struggles here, including mind, body *and* spirit. We draw on transpersonal psychology, a branch of psychology which brings together scientific research and ancient spiritual wisdom.

Crisis is not a bad thing, strange as this might seem. Crisis sparks growth and healing at the personal level, change and evolution at the societal level. Mental health care itself is in crisis. We know that psychiatric reliance on medication is not able to offer any cures. At best it can only hope to control symptoms. And we now have whistle-blowers such as award-winning journalist Robert Whitaker, who have brought to our attention an ethical scandal at the heart of the pharmaceutical industry of such horrific proportions that mental health will never be the same again. His book *Anatomy of an Epidemic: Magic bullets, psychiatric drugs, and the astonishing rise of mental illness in America* won the 2010 Investigative Reporters and Editors (IRE) award as the best investigative journalism book. Whatever anybody makes of his work, and there are many who dispute it, it cannot be ignored.

All this makes the timing ideal for *Coping with a Mental Health Crisis*; all this paves the way for its message to be received and heard. We need a deeper understanding of what mental distress is about, we need a different way of seeing mental health struggles, we need healing approaches that work. You will find all of these here in what I call 'a revisioning of mental health'.

This deeper understanding has long been available but is just now starting to find its way more into the mainstream. In this book I explore trends in mental health and in therapy that are increasingly helping people to make sense of their experience. Some of these trends might once have been dismissed by the medical establishment but have now become mainstream, such as mindfulness, which over the past few years has become a mainstream therapeutic practice. Mindfulness is now taught in such strongholds of convention as the army and the Civil Service. Other therapeutic practices have yet to become integrated into conventional mental health care, and may be new to you or seem unfamiliar, unusual. It is worth keeping an open mind, however, as your crisis may be a call to explore the psyche and your healing in new ways.

Emerging trends

At the very least these emerging trends need to be carefully examined to see what they offer that more conventional medical approaches do not. As well as covering more well-known therapies, this book also looks at some of these emerging approaches. It aims to present information about such trends in a balanced way, so that you are aware of new directions in mental health treatment. This is not to recommend any particular approach, or even to suggest you follow any or all of them, but to report on well-known as well as emerging areas so that you are in a position to make an informed choice about your care.

We desperately need approaches that go beyond medicalizing our experience and that honour our emotional and spiritual needs. Such a stance is nothing new. Back in the 1960s R.D. Laing was one of the first to call for change in the psychiatric profession, which he felt was wrong to treat extreme psychological states as a purely biological phenomenon, without regard for family or cultural influences. Some people feel that things have not moved on significantly since his time – psychiatrist Dr Alan Sanderson, addressing the Royal College of Psychiatrists in London, said, 'Since I qualified as a doctor nearly fifty years ago, there have been tremendous advances in the practice of medicine. Every branch of medicine has been transformed – every branch, that is, except psychiatry . . .'

The crisis within the mental health field is, however, already starting to spark change. The therapeutic approach known as Open Dialogue is rapidly catching on. Open Dialogue, which started in Finland and now exists in this country both as Open Dialogue and as Peer-supported Open Dialogue (POD), aims to support the individual within his or her own network at a time of crisis, with minimal medication. Soteria safe houses, which provide space for people going through acute mental distress, have had a new lease of life in Vermont and Bradford, and there is now a UK Soteria Network. We even have transpersonal psychiatry networks beginning to appear, such as the Vereniging voor Transpersoonlikje Psychiatrie in the Netherlands. Psychiatrists themselves are calling for change, as seen in, for instance, a special article, 'Psychiatry beyond the current paradigm' in the *British Journal of Psychiatry*, to which 29 psychiatrists put their name.[1] Part of a series of articles arguing that psychiatry is in crisis, this calls for psychiatry to move beyond the dominance of the current technological paradigm. The emphasis on psychiatry as 'a brain science' has been too reductionist – and leads to people's core inner needs being ignored, say the authors. 'The increasing focus on neuroscience has meant that other important developments in the provision of care and support for people with mental health problems over the course of the past century have been neglected.'

Each one of us now has an unprecedented opportunity to contribute to this very real change. We can play our part. You can too, by seeking treatment that honours the deeper healing needs of your psyche and soul, by refusing to settle for anything less.

This book

When we're in crisis our first priority has to be staying safe and getting through the worst of the crisis. By the time you're well enough to be reading this book you're hopefully already over the worst. Part 1, 'Revisioning mental health', will help you to start making sense of what you've been through, to find the deeper meaning to your struggles.

It will help you look at mental health from the transpersonal perspective, including some of the possible causes and explanations of your struggles from that viewpoint. Throughout the book I draw on my personal experience, nowhere more so than in Chapter 3, 'Changing our perspective'. There you will find an alternative, transpersonal perspective on certain 'symptoms'. I share some of what I have learnt from personal experience about the relationship between 'madness' and mysticism. I have been privileged to gain insight into the relationship between 'losing our mind' in psychological distress and 'going beyond the mind' in mystical states. This book is unique. I am not unique, though. Many of you have had these experiences. Many of you will recognize yourselves in these pages. This is why I feel compelled to share my experience, to speak my truth, even though it is not easy for me to bare my soul in such a public way.

Part 2 of the book, 'Seven steps to healing', is a call to action. If you want to heal and grow, you will need to be proactive in creating that. The seven steps can't be simply read; they have to be lived. As you begin to take small steps, you will begin to take your life back into your own hands. You will start to feel empowered and that will make you want to do more, take bigger steps, until finally you will have stepped firmly back into the centre of your life, guiding it from the core of your being.

In Part 3, 'Healing approaches', we look at some of the methods you might want to make use of as you engage in the seven steps, from talking therapies to mindfulness, from nutritional medicine to homeopathy. The thorny subject of medication is also covered. This is a small book for the vast range of healing approaches available. Please do not limit yourself to those I have been able to cover. There is such a wealth of therapeutic methods on offer today, including a whole body of excellent work relating to trauma, not included here. What I have aimed to do is give you a taste of just how many options there are.

In the final chapter on healing approaches, I explore different perspectives on mental health from various world traditions under 'Working with soul'. You do not have to take all or any of these on board, but I want to draw your attention to them to show how culturally limited we might be in our understanding of mental health, and to point out elements Western health care might absorb from other disciplines, just as it has absorbed mindfulness, to create integrative, holistic mental health care. My aim is to help you to start thinking outside the 'illness' box. When we're able to drop the 'illness' label, that is when healing and growth become possible.

Part 1
REVISIONING MENTAL HEALTH

1

Finding the deeper meaning

The lino is cold, the wall hard, the staff uninterested. It's 3.00 a.m. I'm sitting on the floor in the corridor, hunched up, leaning against the wall, hugging my legs. The night staff huddle in the office, ignoring me.

This is a very scary place. For a young 20-year-old woman who has led a pretty sheltered life, it's not a nice place to be. People behave in very strange ways and do and say things that I can't make sense of. We have group sessions where I'm too terrified to say a single word in case they decide I've got to stay in this dreadful, surreal hospital even longer.

This is just a snippet of my memories from a very long time ago – 30 years to be precise – when I found myself admitted to an acute psychiatric ward. If you have been through a nightmarish ordeal, if you are struggling to get through each day, I want to reassure you that I know that place. I've been there. Today, however, that past, those memories, seem so far from the happy, fulfilled life I'm living that it is almost as though they belong to someone else, a different person. And in many ways they do. The inner and outer journey I've been on has completely changed who I am and what my priorities are. The healing I've been through has completely transformed my life. Today I teach mindfulness, a form of self-awareness and self-compassion. Of those who attend my groups, many are struggling with mental health issues such as depression, anxiety or post-traumatic stress. I've had the privilege of working with soldiers returning from Iraq and Afghanistan and I've trained UK National Health Service (NHS) therapists.

What is a mental health crisis?

One of the common defining features of a mental health crisis is the sheer intensity of it. It can consume every moment of our day and night, our whole being. Despite certain common features, however, each of us experiences crisis in our own unique, individual way. Here are some aspects you may recognize:

- You may feel completely overwhelmed.
- You may feel unable to cope with everyday tasks like cooking or showering.
- You may experience a rollercoaster of intense emotions, including extreme fear, even terror.
- You may feel isolated and totally alone with what you are or were going through (some feel abandoned by God).
- You may feel desolate and despairing.
- Time may seem to have speeded up or slowed down.
- You may have or have had difficulty sleeping for days or weeks on end.
- You may have or have had strange or worrying physical sensations, such as feelings of energy moving or vibrating through your body.
- You may feel intensely sensitive to everything – light, sound, physical sensations, hot and cold.
- You may find that your thinking feels confused as your rational mind desperately struggles to make sense of what is going on.
- Symbols and coincidences may become significant for you.
- You may have unusual experiences, such as a night-time dream actually happening the following day in a pre-cognitive way.
- You may see unusual or frightening things in your mind's eye; your inner and outer worlds may blur so that it becomes difficult to tell them apart. Indeed, your inner world is likely to take prominence during the crisis.
- You may have flashes of spiritual insight or some experiences that feel profoundly spiritual even if you have never before taken an interest in spirituality or religion.
- You may have a sense of your world as you knew it falling apart.

All of this can be deeply distressing, even excruciating, to go through, but I really want to reassure you that many of us have been through it and gone on to turn our lives around. It has proved to be the catalyst for healing, healing which we maybe didn't even realize was needed: until, that is, the psyche erupted in crisis, like a volcano spewing out all that needs to come to the surface. If you are feeling or experiencing any of this now, or anything else that feels unbearable, please reach out for support. Telling somebody you need help can feel difficult but is essential if you are suffering in any of these ways.

Broadly, then, for the purposes of this book we can define a mental health crisis as any mental state that brings a profound interruption to life as we know it, an overriding feeling of being suddenly removed from all that made life familiar beforehand – routines, work, loved ones, even habits such as listening to music or watching TV. It might be described as an eruption from the unknown, of unrecognized psychic forces within us that, often after years of repression, finally burst their banks and threaten to overwhelm us. There may be a trigger such as losing a job or loved one, falling in love, or reaching mid-life, but these external events may also draw our attention – often dramatically and painfully – to inner states that have been brewing for many years, whose roots perhaps go back to childhood.

Features of a mental health crisis vary from individual to individual and include the range of psychological, emotional and physical characteristics mentioned.

One way of looking at this range of features is as our inner soul calling out for healing. However you define it, a mental health crisis is a wake-up call of the first order, a clarion call that something is wrong. A mental health crisis is a chance to get our profoundest needs met – though it may be very hard to believe at the time.

Unanswered questions

When I sat on that cold linoleum hospital floor it was the summer between my first and second years at university. Something, it seemed, had gone wildly wrong. Why had it happened? How could I make sure this never happened again? I had many unanswered questions. You too may be feeling lost, overwhelmed, confused, maybe even angry, isolated, despairing. You too may have many unanswered questions.

'Sometimes it's best not to try to understand these things,' I was told by the psychiatrist when I asked for counselling or psychotherapy. Today that approach seems ostrich-like to say the least. How can we heal our deep wounds if we don't try to understand them? Fortunately, I did find the answers I was looking for, but it took 20 years.

My hope with this book is to save you much unnecessary suffering and much time, to present information that will help you make informed choices. Informed readers make for empowered patients, as well as carers and supporters. This empowerment is the basis of our 'Seven steps to healing'. I will be presenting a different way of looking at mental health, different from the classic 'illness' approach, and I will be giving you clear guidance on the seven steps to successful healing. I want you to know that, like me, you can get through what may feel like the most challenging period of your life. Many others have too. Like all of us, you can come through to a whole new level, living a happier and healthier life.

A parallel perspective

Ursula has been forcibly held. She has been held under the Mental Health Act, sectioned, and she has been held down by four staff, wielding needles, injecting her with anti-psychotics. She has been hospitalized ten times in all.

Ursula had been written off by the medical profession. She could easily have ended up withdrawn, not being able to function socially, not able to work, not able to sustain an intimate relationship. Instead, Ursula is now living a fulfilling and fulfilled life: married, a loving partner, a gorgeous little daughter, making a contribution to her community through her work, writing and speaking. Ursula has turned her life around because of a choice she made: the choice to focus on healing and growth, not on illness and symptoms. She shares her inspiring story in Part 2.

We can change our perspective at any moment we choose. We can buy into the story 'this diagnosis is for life' or we can buy into 'this diagnosis means there is healing work to do'. Simply how we choose to frame our experiences, the lens we choose to see them through, can and will make all the difference. Have you ever seen one of those black and white images that present an optical illusion? At first all you can see is a vase. If you're told there's another image there and you look longer, softening your gaze, you see a parallel image, two faces looking at each other (see Figure 1). At first it's difficult to see the second image, the alternative perspective, but if we've been told it's there, we can keep looking until we too can

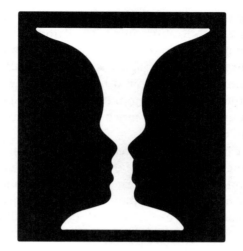

Figure 1

see it. Once we've spotted the alternative perspective it seems so obvious we don't know why we couldn't see it before.

We can only reframe our experiences as Ursula and others have and see them from this broader, more positive, more healing perspective, if we know such an alternative is available. Like the optical illusion, we will only look for and see the parallel image if someone says it is there. Otherwise we won't even know, we won't even think, to look for it.

In the process of making sense of what is happening, we can find a deeper meaning to our suffering, to our struggles. What at first may seem an appalling disaster can in fact, when we look more closely, turn out to be a blessing in disguise, the prompt we needed to look at what isn't working in our lives, what needs changing. Such a huge upheaval can be a signal that learning and healing are needed, that growth and change is the only positive way forward.

Embracing mind, body *and* spirit

The information you will find here comes from the transpersonal field, 'trans' meaning 'beyond' the personal. The transpersonal is a model or world view which goes beyond everyday reality, beyond ordinary experience, to encompass a wider understanding of the cosmos. This is a holistic approach, embracing not only mind and body but spirit as well. Why might it be helpful to include spirit, the spiritual dimension, in our search for deeper meaning? Many of our significant concerns are highly spiritual without us necessarily realizing it. Our need to love and be loved, our need for purpose in our lives, our need for community, all are spiritual issues. These kinds of concern tend to be much more alive for us in times of crisis, in times of ill health.

When we're looking for the deeper meaning, we need to turn our attention to the bigger picture. The transpersonal offers us this bigger picture. It has long provided a far greater, deeper understanding of the causes of mental distress than conventional psychiatry seems able to do. Some mental health professionals are willing to acknowledge this gap in understanding within the mainstream. American Surgeon General David Satcher admitted in his *Mental Health: A report of the Surgeon General, 1999*, 'the precise causes [etiologies] of mental disorders are not known'. I might add 'are not known *within mainstream psychiatry*'. And so, in our search for deeper meaning, we find ourselves turning to a field which acknowledges the mystery of life, which allows for the numinous, which allows for suffering to be a vehicle to healing and growth: the transpersonal field.

This kind of information may be totally new to you. Please bear with me, however. Like Christopher Columbus setting out across the oceans to explore the world, you too are setting out on a journey, a healing journey, not knowing what to expect or what you might find. The approaches I cover can be a map for you to begin to find your way across the unknown waters to the destination you seek. As I said earlier, you do not have to take on board everything these approaches suggest. It's good to keep a questioning, enquiring frame of mind, testing the information out for yourself. I do feel, however, that the core messages of these perspectives should be examined carefully, as they offer clues as to what may be missing in established psychiatric wisdom, and what so many people are seeking.

So what is the transpersonal field? How can it offer insight into our particular mental health struggles? How can the transpersonal help us find the deeper meaning of our distress? We'll answer these questions in the next chapter, as we focus on transpersonal psychology and its view of breakdown as potential breakthrough.

2

Transpersonal psychology

Double-binds

Damned if you do, damned if you don't. Double-binds were the subject of R.D. Laing's book *Sanity, Madness and the Family* in 1964. R.D. Laing was known for his strong views on mental 'illness', which questioned assumptions about the biological basis of schizophrenia and explored the influence of unconscious family dynamics on psychosis. He once described insanity as 'a perfectly rational response to an insane world'. Through his research, Laing showed how some parents unwittingly create double-bind scenarios for their children, somehow far worse than lose–lose situations. He also showed how such double-binds can create 'psychotic' symptoms in those who are presented with intolerable Catch-22 situations in their daily lives. I came across this book many years ago, when I was trying to work out why I'd ended up in hospital.

My story
The double-bind for me came from my parents being very unhappily married and at odds with one another. To love my mother was a betrayal of my father. To love my father was a betrayal of my mother. One way a child in this situation will cope is by creating an internal split. By doing so, the developing ego avoids greater damage.

The dysfunction in my family was intensified by my father being an alcoholic. So I had the added complication of both loving him deeply and, because of his abusive behaviour, hating him with a vengeance. At the time I was too young to understand that he was carrying his own deep, unaddressed wounds. Such strong, totally contrasting emotions are not easy for a child to hold or to cope with, especially when the family doesn't know how to talk about feelings at all.

When my parents finally split up, I too split up, split apart. Later, with the help of psychotherapy, it wasn't difficult for me to see how the whole edifice of my psyche had come crashing down at that time. As Rumi, the mystic poet, says, it is through the wound that the Light enters. I was catapulted into a profound psychospiritual crisis, such was the severe wounding I carried which needed tending.

Today I see that spell in hospital as the beginning of my healing journey, of realizing that my psyche was calling out for help. That period of crisis turned out to be just the beginning of a whole process of deep transformation. Laing's research was enormously helpful for me. His book was my first taste of finding the deeper meaning in mental distress.

What is transpersonal psychology?

Transpersonal psychology is a school of psychology which goes beyond the personal to include the transcendental, the interconnectedness of all beings. It brings together ancient spiritual wisdom and understanding with modern scientific research, using psychological methods to explore our spiritual life and experiences. It is an established, recognized academic field. From the perspective of transpersonal psychology, mental health crises can be seen as periods of deep transformation with the potential to help us grow and heal. This is obviously enormously helpful in our search for deeper meaning and a positive way forward.

The origins of transpersonal psychology

Transpersonal psychology grew out of humanistic psychology and the work of American psychologist Abraham Maslow. He is best known for his theory on the hierarchy of needs, a scale of needs humans fulfil on their way to optimum psychological health, as well as his research into peak experiences. Maslow felt that current psychiatry was too reductionist and clinical, focusing too much on symptoms and not enough on human growth and potential.

During the 1960s, Maslow, along with others including Stanislav Grof and Viktor Frankl, started meeting in California. Grof, a psychiatrist from Czechoslovakia, has been influential, along with his wife Christina, in shaping transpersonal psychology, coining the term 'spiritual emergency'. Frankl, an Austrian neurologist and psychiatrist, was a Holocaust survivor and the author of *Man's Search for Meaning*. This group felt that psychology was missing an important dimension: that aspect of human experience which transcends the individual or personal. The pre-personal was being acknowledged, the period when an infant has not yet grasped a sense of being a separate individual, as was the personal, when the ego is fully formed. But what these psychologists and psychiatrists were interested in was human experience beyond the personal, states of consciousness beyond the ego: the transpersonal.

A new movement, that of transpersonal psychology, was born, accompanied by an Association for Transpersonal Psychology and an academic periodical, the *Journal of Transpersonal Psychology*.

Although transpersonal psychology grew directly out of humanistic psychology, its roots go back further. Its development owes a great deal to the work of Carl Jung, and William James before him, at the turn of the twentieth century. In those early days, psychology as an academic subject was in its infancy. James, described as 'one of the great pioneers of psychology' by Andrew Powell and Chris MacKenna,[2] was the first to attempt to investigate and classify the relationship between psychology and spirituality. In his work *The Varieties of Religious Experience* (published in 1902) James argued that it is not possible to understand profound spiritual experiences at the cognitive, intellectual level; they are ineffable and have to be personally experienced to be understood.

This fledgling interest in the scientific research of human consciousness and spirituality was swept away with the rise in popularity of Freud's essentially atheistic approach to psychology. As Russell Shorto tellingly narrates in his book *Saints and Madmen*, 'Freud, after pondering a friend's description of religiosity as an "oceanic feeling", famously remarked "I cannot discover this 'oceanic' feeling in myself"'.[3] This was precisely James's point, that such numinous states have to be personally experienced to be understood. Freud had not experienced them. This was the distinction between Freud and Jung, his contemporary. Jung went through a long period of psychospiritual crisis, along with profound spiritual experiences and insight which informed his entire body of work. He understood unitive states of consciousness, the 'oceanic', in a way that Freud didn't.

Jung, however, was ahead of his time, and the prominent trend, with Freud leading the way, was 'medical materialism', as James called it. It was not until the second half of the twentieth century, as we have seen, that the scientific exploration of consciousness beyond the individual really became established as a field in its own right. In the ferment of the 1960s other key players who challenged orthodox psychology and psychiatry, aligning themselves with the transpersonal, were R.D. Laing, the Scottish psychiatrist, and John Weir Perry, the American Jungian psychiatrist. As Shorto puts it: 'By looking at psychosis as a mere illness, these thinkers said, psychiatry misses the whole point of the affliction: that it is ultimately an attempt to find deeper meaning'.[4]

The healing potential of crisis

The clinical findings of Jung, Grof, Laing and Perry all led them to draw similar conclusions: that a period of mental health crisis could be seen as the psyche's attempt to heal itself. Jung talked about the process of 'individuation', where Maslow used the expression 'self-actualization'. Laing thought in terms of 'the reintegration of personality'; Perry saw it as a natural process of 'renewal'; Grof found that spiritual emergency could lead to spiritual emergence, a process of healing and awakening. If correctly understood and supported, such crises held enormous potential.

Both Laing and Perry received research grants to study alternatives to acute inpatient settings. They set up residential units in their respective countries and kept the use of medication to a minimum. Perry's take on this was that it suppressed the deep contents of the psyche and was not conducive to healing. This was precisely Dr Daniel Dorman's view when working therapeutically with Cathy Penney, who has written the Foreword to this book.

Still today, particularly skilled and wise psychiatrists will not automatically prescribe psychiatric drugs if they feel a patient will benefit more without them. Often these clinicians are also psychotherapists and thus tend to have more insight into the potential for human suffering to be the gateway to real and lasting healing. Psychiatrist Paul Fleischman is one example. Fleischman's book *The Healing Spirit: Explorations in religion and psychotherapy* won him the Oskar Pfister Award for 'important contributions to the humanistic and spiritual side of psychiatric issues' in 1993. 'He believes in the fifty-minute session . . . prescribes Prozac where he thinks it helpful and resists patients who ask for drugs when he thinks it won't be helpful'.[5]

Defining transpersonal psychology

Definitions of transpersonal psychology do vary, but researchers Denise Lajoie and Sam Shapiro have suggested that there are five key factors. Lajoie and Shapiro, in the *Journal of Transpersonal Psychology*, reviewed 40 definitions of transpersonal psychology in the academic literature from 1968 to 1991 and found that the five major themes were:

- states of consciousness
- higher or ultimate potential
- beyond the ego or personal self
- transcendence
- the spiritual.

As a result, the authors proposed this definition: 'Transpersonal Psychology is concerned with the study of humanity's highest potential, and with the recognition, understanding, and realization of unitive, spiritual, and transcendent states of consciousness.'

Breakdown or breakthrough?

In a slightly later book, *The Politics of Experience*, Laing addresses more transpersonal or spiritual themes such as the dissolution or transcendence of the ego. We can intentionally seek this through meditation and spiritual practices or it can happen spontaneously. The 'mad' person, Laing argued, finds him- or herself unwittingly catapulted into this process and will flounder without the right guidance.

It was, however, in the work of the Grofs where, much later, I came across the term 'spiritual emergency'. While we normally develop emotionally, psychologically and spiritually in a gradual way, sometimes this process of growth can speed up and tip over into crisis. Spiritual emergency, or psychospiritual crisis, is essentially a process of profound inner transformation.

I felt a huge relief as I read about the overlap between transcendent, mystical experiences and the experience of those going through mental breakdown. The transpersonal research suggested that with the right support the psyche could come through such periods of psychospiritual crisis. Such a crisis had the potential to be healing and regenerative; it could be a breakthrough to a whole new level of wellness and functioning.

As I delved deeper into the transpersonal psychology literature I found the related idea, in the work of John Weir Perry, that psychospiritual crisis or spiritual emergency can be seen as a natural process of renewal. The psyche needs to be allowed and supported to go through this disorganization on its way to reorganization. In his book *Trials of the Visionary Mind*, Perry wrote, 'the psyche is striving to dismantle [the] previous self in order to reorganize it along new lines' but 'the person is caught between opposite pressures: one from the psyche to go through disorganization on the way to reorganization, and the other from the psychiatric system to put a stop to that and get back to "normal"'.[6]

The right understanding and support are, therefore, crucial. Without them the disintegrating ego is very vulnerable and may not manage the journey back to health. In an ideal world, this would be provided by some kind of safe haven where sensitively trained staff or those with personal experience of extreme states would support rather than restrain or drug. John Weir Perry founded Diabasis in San Francisco, California, in 1970. On similar lines to Soteria (see page 111), Diabasis was conceived as a safe place for people going through a first psychotic breakdown to process their experience with minimal medication and with loving support from staff. 'There was a consensus on the basic viewpoint that the acute 'psychotic' episode under discussion typically contains elements of a spontaneous reorganizing of the self and that therefore, if it is handled well, this may result in self-healing'.[7] In reporting Diabasis research outcomes, Dr Perry says, 'Our most surprising finding in the cases of early acute episode was that grossly "psychotic" clients have usually come into a coherent and reality-oriented state spontaneously within two to six days, without need for medications'.[8] Or, to put it another way, 'People would come in just as crazy as could be on the first day or two, but they'd settle down very soon into a state of coherency and clarity . . . The calming effect of a supportive environment is truly amazing!' Perry concluded that schizophrenia can be a self-healing process – one in which the pathological complexes can dissolve themselves.[9]

As we shall see, this is precisely what Open Dialogue therapists are finding: given the support and opportunity, clients experience spontaneous recovery.

My story – the Spiritual Crisis Network

Unfortunately, during that first period of crisis, the natural process was interrupted for me by the trauma of hospitalization and thwarted by the heavy use of medication. I spent most of my second year of university in bed, heavily sedated. It was 20 years before I was able to re-engage with the process and move through to the all-important phase of reorganization. That was in 2003, during a trip to Egypt. This time I went through psychospiritual crisis in a more conscious way; my experience was completely different from that first time. I was supported and validated by those around me and, although the crisis was far more severe, I didn't end up in hospital. I did end up in a wheelchair for a few days because my legs gave way with the shock of what I was going through emotionally and psychologically.

A year later, I organized the first of three residential conferences on spiritual emergency, calling the series 'Revisioning Mental Health'. From there I set up, with like-minded others, the Spiritual Crisis Network, which has become a registered charity. And I went on to write my first book, *In Case of Spiritual Emergency*. Such is the potential of these crises when understood and supported.

An academic field

Today, transpersonal psychology is an established academic field which draws on spiritual wisdom from many different traditions. It explores and explains psychospiritual development, from our deepest scars to our highest potential, from our crises to our enlightenment. This is a model or a way of looking at the world that understands the spiritual and that makes use of ancient sacred knowledge, integrating it into modern psychological research and theory. The *International Journal of Transpersonal Studies* (*IJTS*) is a double-blind peer-reviewed journal which publishes the latest in-depth studies, while the *Journal of Transpersonal Research* also publishes research in the field. Some universities offer degree programmes in transpersonal psychology, such as Northampton University's MSc in Transpersonal Psychology and Consciousness Studies or the master's degree at Sofia University (formerly the Institute of Transpersonal Psychology) in California. A key professional body is the Association for Transpersonal Psychology (ATP) and the British Psychological Society also has a Transpersonal Section.

In this chapter we have covered the essence of the transpersonal approach. We have seen how a mental health crisis has the potential to be a breakthrough rather than a breakdown, and how this more positive and creative view is increasingly gaining acceptance. Let's now take a closer look at some of the detail of actual experiences, at some of the symptoms. Viewing these from the transpersonal perspective forms part of the revisioning of mental health, our theme throughout this section.

3

Changing our perspective

Remember the parallel images of the black and white optical illusion? (See page 17.) There doesn't have to be just one way of looking at things. In this chapter we're going to take another look at the parallel, alternative take on mental health. We're going to look at some of the symptoms; they take on a whole new meaning when we change our perspective.

Bipolar states

Bipolar states are characterized by manic highs and depressive lows, which is why they used to be called manic-depression. A personal account of living with this is Kay Redfield Jamison's *An Unquiet Mind*. A psychiatrist herself (Professor of Psychiatry at Johns Hopkins University School of Medicine) and a co-author of the standard medical text on bipolar states, Jamison approaches her struggles very much from the mainstream biomedical perspective. With the additional understanding of psychospiritual processes, we can shed further light on what she describes.

Mythological themes

In one passage, Jamison writes about her mind being 'drenched in awful sounds and images of decay and dying'. This is very typical for someone going through psychospiritual crisis. Archetypal themes of death and decay are very much present at times of psychological renewal. As John Weir Perry says: 'Whenever a profound experience of change is about to take place, its harbinger is the motif of death. The question why is not particularly mysterious, since it is the limited view and appraisal of oneself that primarily must be outgrown.'[10]

The ego can experience this renewal process as a death of itself, albeit usually temporarily. It is the death of our old self, our old beliefs, our old way of being in the world. Although the process is one of psychological 'death' rather than physical death, often we can have a very real sense and fear of our impending actual death. Death followed by new birth is thus a universal theme. To label such images as pathological, as indicative of 'illness', is to dismiss our psyche's way of communicating.

Some schools of Buddhism positively encourage meditating on the themes of death and decay, in order to understand the law of impermanence, that nothing is permanent, that everything ultimately changes, decays or dies. If we understand death and dying as part of the never-ending cycle of life and understand that the ego too can 'die' we can respond differently to it. This level of insight helps us to make sense of the horrors we are going through.

Birth and death, creation and destruction, good versus evil: these are the timeless, mythological themes characteristic of psychospiritual crisis. If they go unrecognized and unacknowledged, they are likely to come back again and again with a vengeance until they are seen for what they are: messages of hope and healing. The alternative is that they are medicated into submission for good, never to illuminate or communicate with us again.

Creativity and mania

A number of famous artists and writers are thought to have suffered from bipolar states. For example, one of the most public figures in the UK to suffer from this creative mania and suicidal depression is the writer and broadcaster Stephen Fry. He has spoken publicly about his experience, which was depicted in the documentary *Stephen Fry: The secret life of the manic depressive*.

Why is it that artists and creatives should particularly suffer from this combination of mania and depression? The transpersonal literature sheds light on this. American author Julia Cameron's book *The Artist's Way: A spiritual path to higher creativity* has sold four million copies worldwide. She gives an answer in the first few pages. She sees creative energy and spiritual energy as one and the same. The same life force that creates newborn babies and springtime lambs also creates beautiful works of art and bestselling books. Cameron is not alone in equating creative energy with life force, spiritual energy.

Elaine Aron, author of *The Highly Sensitive Person*, explains part of the challenge for creatives. Highly Sensitive People (HSPs) – and most creatives are – need plenty of quiet time. The complete contrast between the withdrawal and isolation of the creative process and the very public, stimulating and, for HSPs, often overwhelming promotion of the work 'out in the world' can be very difficult to navigate.

So when creative energy comes pouring through in a bout of mania, one way of seeing it is as spiritual energy, energy which needs grounding, energy seeking an outlet. Many find it very helpful to draw, paint, sculpt or write as a way of channelling and processing this energy. Failure to ground it can leave us overwhelmed and at its mercy.

Understanding mania as energy does not necessarily make it any easier to ground. I certainly don't want to minimize or glamorize the suffering which can come with each bout. It does mean, though, that we can reframe it, putting it in a different context rather than merely pathologizing it as a 'symptom of illness'.

Everyday activities which can be grounding include:

- cooking, such as kneading bread
- physical exercise, especially walking in nature
- housework, hoovering, cleaning the bathroom, etc.
- gardening, like digging or weeding
- physical contact, such as massage
- DIY, decorating, sanding, painting, etc.

On a symbolic or metaphoric level, with the planting of bulbs or planting out of seedlings, nature's growth can mirror our own psychological growth. Equally, we can do housework and cleaning holding in mind the idea of cleansing ourselves at the same time as our home. For a full discussion of grounding techniques see my book *In Case of Spiritual Emergency*.

Depression

With the intensity of this fiery energy, of needing to go for ten-mile runs to discharge it, of hardly sleeping for days or weeks on end and not eating properly, it is not difficult to see how the body and mind might collapse, exhausted, burnt out, depressed. The body above all needs rest, recuperation and dietary supplements to replenish all its drained natural reserves. As you recuperate you need regular, nourishing meals. Ask for help with shopping or cooking if you need it. Trust your instinct with what foods your body needs, as long as that feels healthy. Rest and relax as much as possible through the day – give yourself permission to do so in order to help yourself recover. Balance that with gentle exercise; get out in nature as much as you can.

Dark night of the soul

The dark night of the soul is a journey experienced by many during a crisis. This dark time, described by sixteenth-century Spanish mystic Saint John of the Cross, by Saint Thérèse of Lisieux and by Mother Teresa of Calcutta in her letters, can be one of the most profound challenges to anyone struggling with a mental health crisis. Today, psychospiritual writers such as Stephanie Sorrell, author of *Depression as a Spiritual Journey*, speak about depression as going through a 'dark night of the soul'. A 'dark night' is characterized by feelings of loss and confusion. We can feel abandoned by God. There can be accompanying depression as we experience an emptying of the self, as psychiatrist Dr Gerald May puts it. An American prisons psychiatrist and theologian, Dr May is the author of *The Dark Night of the Soul: A psychiatrist explores the connection between darkness and spiritual growth*. In this he argues that the 'shadow' side of the spiritual life is a vital and integral part of true growth and healing. 'Superficial and naively upbeat spirituality does not heal and enrich the soul,' he warns – though his message is that the dark night is not necessarily a time of unending suffering and despair but a time of deep transition.

Often it seems to be a gradual process, with each period of depression followed by a renewed sense of clarity and purpose as each layer of the wounded self is peeled away. This can be seen as a progressive cleansing and purification, making way for something better, allowing us to function at a higher, fuller level. After all the suffering and confusion of the dark night, this is the new dawn. The important thing, argues Dr May, is to support the psychospiritual process while treating the depression in the most appropriate way.

Psychosis and schizophrenia

The relationship between mental health and spirituality, between 'madness' and mysticism, is extremely complex. It is also a very loaded issue for many and can often be difficult for mental health professionals or family members to begin to grasp. This is especially so for those whose world view is essentially secular. From the transpersonal perspective, when we look at some of the symptoms of conditions such as 'psychosis' or 'schizophrenia', we see something very different happening: we see the parallel image of the optical illusion.

Understanding 'delusions'

A colleague once had to persuade someone not to throw himself off the top of a ten-storey building, thinking he could fly. This is obviously very dangerous; anyone going through this needs a great deal of support and needs to be kept safe. It is, however, worth exploring why someone might think they could fly. When I was first in crisis at the age of 20 I too remember being in touch with that part of us that *can* move through time and space, that can 'fly'. In the process of being broken open by the psychospiritual crisis I was going through, I was becoming directly in touch with my soul for the first time ever. The locus had shifted so that I was more identified with the spiritual than with this physical body called Catherine. This is my understanding of why a person might think he could fly, but for those who have not had such direct contact with their soul it may well be difficult to grasp.

This strong identification with spirit and loss of connection with our physical bodies can pose very real dangers to some people. Others might think they can breathe under water or walk through flames. While we need to do everything necessary to keep that person safe, at least we can begin to understand why he or she might think that way.

Our true mind is experienced as inner stillness and silence: deep peace. The endless inner chatter is gone. My experience of such awakened states, on the few occasions I've touched into them, is that the mind can feel spacious, empty, even blank. There are simply no thoughts arising. On one occasion as I moved into such a state I also had a sense of thoughts falling away, of slipping out of the mind, out of my grasp, leaving an inner emptiness, spaciousness and silence. This can be very disconcerting: a feeling of not being able to think in the usual sense, almost as if our minds are literally emptying.

Anyone plunged into psychospiritual crisis having this kind of experience is likely to find it terrifying. It is easy to see how we might experience it as our mind *being* emptied. Our tendency is to believe that somebody outside of us, external to us, must be doing it.

In a desperate attempt to explain it, we might describe it as someone taking our thoughts or controlling our thoughts. As a society, we have so little understanding of the process of spiritual development, of spiritual awakening, that we neither know how to recognize, describe nor make sense of such states. During psychospiritual crisis the situation is further complicated by all our wounding coming to the surface. The title of psychiatrist Dr Russell Razzaque's book says it all: *Breaking Down is Waking Up*.

Hallucinations or visions?

As a child, 'Sally had recurring visions of flames licking around her bed and the red face of the devil would appear at night and in her dreams'. Not surprising when we hear she had a fundamentalist schoolteacher who terrified the seven-year-old 'with threats of hell and damnation'. 'In adulthood Sally seemed to overcome these fears but, following major surgery, which left her body scarred, she once again succumbed to these visions, living from day to day in a state of sheer panic.'[11]

Sally was one of Dr Andrew Powell's patients and he shares her story in his chapter on 'Soul-centered psychotherapy' in *Spiritism and Mental Health*. From the transpersonal perspective, the important thing with any such 'symptoms', whether hearing voices, seemingly irrational thinking or seeing visions, is to put them in their context. Out of context, Sally would come across as an adult who was having irrational hallucinations. In context, her experiences make complete sense. A practitioner with the right training and psychospiritual understanding could help her, as indeed Dr Powell was able to do.

I find the story of what happened to Carl Jung in this context fascinating. In 1913 he had horrific visions of Europe flooded in blood with thousands of bodies drowned in that bloodbath. As a psychiatrist, he thought he was hallucinating and feared he was heading for 'psychosis', only to see his visions come true with the outbreak of the First World War.

Sometimes when people describe their symptoms it seems as if the boundary between them and the spirit world is not strong enough, as if the veil is too thin. In that case we can learn psychic protection.

Paul contacted me looking for support and guidance. He described some of what he had experienced which had resulted in him being diagnosed as mentally ill. He had seen spirits, dead people, walking around and had many other experiences which had really frightened and disturbed him. Now he was gradually reducing the medication he was on but was very concerned about coming off completely in case he re-experienced such horrors. One possible route for Paul would be to learn psychic protection so that he could strengthen the boundary between himself and the spirit world. First, Paul would need to acknowledge the spirit world as real. As long as he held on to the conviction there was no such thing, he would believe his mind had created the 'hallucinations', a terrifying thought for anybody.

Delusions of reference or messages from the Universe?

Another common experience considered a classic feature or 'symptom' of psychosis and schizophrenia is when a person feels he or she is getting messages, for example from the television, radio or billboards. Again, here is a parallel take on this from the transpersonal perspective: author Denise Linn writes that we are surrounded by myriad messages from the Universe, Source or God at all times. Of native American descent, Linn has written *Signposts*, a comprehensive guide to the signs and symbols that come to us from the Universe and how to interpret them. In many ways it is reminiscent of Jungian symbolism. Much of the time, our minds filter most of these out because they would be too overwhelming for us. So whether we see the messages as coming from our own unconscious, from our Higher Self or from Spirit, they can indeed be very helpful.

The difficulty when we are in psychospiritual crisis can be that we lose the ability to filter them out and the sheer volume becomes completely overwhelming. At the same time we can be swirling in a vortex of fear, past trauma and deep wounding, all escalating into terror. As we project this out on to the world, the effect is that the messages mirror back to us, taking on a threatening, menacing tone. Before we know it, we are in the grip of paranoia. Understanding such psychological processes can be an enormous help.

Over the years I have fine-tuned my ability to read the messages. This is a skill we can acquire. I now do my best to be open to them when they come, in whatever form; very often for me it's in the lyrics of songs. Recently I found myself spontaneously singing 'We're off to see the wizard, the wonderful wizard of Oz.' This may or may not mean there is a trip to Australia coming up. I like to keep an open mind.

Seeming 'delusions of reference' can manifest in other ways too. Anybody who has experiences similar to the following will understand why so-called schizophrenics might feel people are talking about them.

My story

I was feeling that I had been neglecting my spiritual practice, that if I truly wanted to 'wake up' fully then I needed to spend a lot of time on retreat. I had started to plan when and where I could go on long retreats. I was also aware, though, that this book would be coming out later in the year and I would need to be very much 'out in the world' and visible. There was a lot of work to do. One early morning, as I wrestled with these conflicting needs, I was at the swimming pool. There was only one other woman in the changing rooms. As I put my things in a locker, a metal thermos mug fell out of my bag on to the ceramic tiled floor, making a resounding and very loud 'clang'. I simply said 'Sorry' and put it back in my bag. The other woman replied, 'Don't worry, I'm awake enough.' In that instant I had an 'aha!' moment. I felt reassured that I was already 'awake enough' for the task ahead of me. Yes, going on retreat would nourish and feed me at the soul level, but I needn't worry, I was 'awake enough'.

This example may not sound very significant, but the crucial element is the word 'I'. It refers to the Centre, Source or God. Once we have understood at an experiential level the truth that we are all interconnected, that we are all One, we are all the Centre, we will have experiences in which others appear to speak on our behalf, experiences which in the psychiatric context are called 'delusions of reference'. Over the years I have become more and more attuned to hearing this. I call it 'hearing Spirit' because I am at a loss to know what language to use to describe it. We could equally call it 'touching into the Whole' based on what psychiatrist Dr Russell Razzaque writes in *Breaking Down is Waking Up*.

He shows clearly and simply how the ego creates the illusion of separation, the illusion that we are all separate from one another and from everything around us. He also explains in layman's terms how quantum physics has proved the exact opposite to be true. Advances in science have shown what spiritual masters have known for thousands of years, that the entire universe is a single unified Whole. Every single cell, atom or particle impacts on every other cell, atom and particle. The full implications of this are vast and difficult to conceive. As Razzaque says, 'We now sit on a precipice in which an entirely new understanding of reality can be used to solve all manner of problems from the ecological to the economic, and from the sociological to the psychiatric.'

I hope my experience of 'touching into the Whole' will encourage many others who experience the same thing to speak out. That way we can have a different, parallel conversation about what is happening when someone thinks people are talking about them; that person may be 'touching into the Whole' but have no idea how to cope with that. To complicate matters further, part of what is being mirrored back is likely to be her own fearful projections, her own wounded shadow material. She will feel she is coming under attack from 'outside' and needs to learn to distinguish between the two.

Hearing voices

There are many different reasons for hearing voices. Traditional psychiatry describes hearing voices as 'auditory hallucinations' which are considered a symptom of schizophrenia, but research shows that hearing voices is relatively common and that the majority of people who hear voices do not have mental health issues. Hearing voices may be triggered by, among other things, extreme emotional states, stress or trauma, physical illness, epileptic seizure, bereavement and spiritual experience. Of the many different explanations for this particular symptom, the following case study illustrates the power of suppressed rage to trigger voices.

A psychotherapist tells the story of a mother and daughter. We'll call them Mrs Jones and her daughter Judith. Mrs Jones got in touch with the therapist, asking him to see Judith. She had been hearing voices telling her to kill her mother. He agreed to meet Mrs Jones at the start of the session before seeing Judith. When he met Mrs Jones he described her as one of the most obnoxious women he had ever met, which presumably meant she was also very wounded. He actually felt like being physically violent and had murderous feelings towards her, wanting to put his hands around her neck and throttle her. Fortunately for his reputation and practice, however, he managed to be polite and civil. When she left and Judith came in, during their conversation the therapist shared with Judith the thoughts and feelings he had had towards her mother. That single session was enough for the voices Judith had been hearing, telling her to kill her mother, to stop. Judith was able to begin owning her suppressed rage towards her mother.

The point is that, once we open our minds and explore the alternatives, we do not have to resort to a reductionist and narrowing medicalization of people's experiences which, in therapeutic and life terms, gets them nowhere. While the medical stance undoubtedly has its place, the more we look at some of the 'symptoms' of mania, depression, psychosis or schizophrenia, the more we can see that there is room for parallel explanations which yield more meaning to those going through such experiences. The longer we are willing to look at the vase in the optical illusion, the more likely we are to see the other image, the other perspective, emerging. The more we can hold both views simultaneously, the more we will be able to stop labelling, pathologizing and medicating; the more we will be able to start understanding, supporting and healing.

Under all the emotional and psychological wounding, all the horrific trauma, all the post-traumatic stress, all the severely damaged egos and personalities – underneath it all, there is health longing to emerge, longing to be freed. In the same way that our physical bodies naturally want to move towards healing, so too do our psyches. In the same way that our bodies can be supported to do so, bones mending, scars healing over, so too can our minds.

In Part 2, 'Seven steps to healing', we're going to look at how to go about putting this healing journey into practice in very real, practical terms. These seven steps are full of common sense. They are do-able and achievable. Yet at the same time they are radical and life-changing. You need nothing less than that for your healing. You need to be prepared to stop at nothing, to do whatever it takes to heal. Get ready to take the reins!

Part 2
SEVEN STEPS TO HEALING

Step 1

Taking responsibility

'I had to believe in myself when no one else did.'

Louise

You can heal. I believe totally and utterly in that. Every crisis holds the potential for our personal transformation; every breakdown is potentially more of a breakthrough to a whole new level of wellness and functioning. We know, though, that this potential for healing and growth is by no means always achieved. Our psychiatric hospitals and doctors' surgeries are kept busy with people who have not experienced this.

So how do we fulfil that potential? What does it take? By way of answer I've identified 'Seven steps to healing'. You can think of these as your strategies for success. We need to put certain conditions in place, and following these steps will enable you to do that. We don't expect plants to blossom in our garden if we don't water them, prune them or weed them. They need certain conditions to grow, to bloom. We too have some watering, pruning and weeding to do before we can blossom.

The 'Seven steps to healing' are:

1 taking responsibility
2 reaching out
3 finding the right healthcare professionals
4 focusing on success stories
5 doing away with the toxic
6 making life changes
7 seeing crisis as a gift.

The very first step is taking responsibility for our own healing. All the other steps build on this fundamental cornerstone.

How willing are we?

To take responsibility for our healing we need to do a bit of soul searching. This might sound like an odd question, but how much do we really want to heal? How far are we prepared to go to turn our lives around? Are we willing to truly take responsibility for our own journey to wellness? Medical intuitive and author Caroline Myss illustrates the challenge in the following passage from her book *Why People Don't Heal and How They Can*. It is a thought-provoking account of how we sometimes unconsciously limit ourselves.

Armed with the knowledge of my own resistance to the journey of healing, I decided to ask the participants of a subsequent workshop how important becoming healthy was to them. At first, everyone responded enthusiastically that nothing stood in the way of achieving this goal. But they answered so quickly and so ardently that I knew something was wrong; their response had been mental, not authentic and emotional. The emotional level reveals our true feelings.

I decided to test them by asking them to be specific about the possible changes in lifestyle that they would be willing to make in order to heal . . . I asked the group a series of questions, ratcheting up the level of commitment with each one.

'If healing required changing your job, would you do it?' Most of the members replied yes.

'If healing required moving to another part of the country, would you do it?' Again, most replied yes.

'If healing required that you change most of your attitudes toward others and yourself, would you do so?' Now the group became more selective, pondering with a bit more thought. The responses varied this time, with some saying that they didn't think their attitudes needed that much changing. Others said that if such a level of change were needed, they would give it a try.

. . . 'If healing your emotional and psychological nature required that you experience a physical [or mental] illness, perhaps a long and difficult one, as the means of contact with these parts of yourself, would you accept that challenge?' The majority answered no. Some said they might if they had no other choice. Only one replied, 'Absolutely.'

'If the goal of becoming healthy required you to lose everything familiar to you – home, spouse, job, what then would you say?' This time the group fell silent.

. . . My point in asking these questions, I told them, was neither to scare them nor to make the journey to health look like a bed of hot coals. It was to illustrate that we hold within us – whether or not we realize it – the terms upon which we will move forward with our lives, including the goal of healing an illness.[12]

The reality is, of course, that some people do lose everything, their jobs, their homes and their partners, when going through psycho-spiritual crisis. It can be hard, very hard, at the time and often we have no choice. The Universe strips away all that needs to go, radically pruning away the dead wood, whether we think it is ready for the bonfire or not. If, however, we are able to engage with the steps I outline here, then invariably this leads to whole new growth, to a whole new quality of life.

Our motivation

Ironically, the more we are suffering the more motivated we will probably be to find ways out of that suffering. This has certainly been my experience when teaching mindfulness. Those students in the most emotional and psychological pain are those who are most motivated to do the home practice. This means they really learn the mindfulness and fully benefit from it. They are the ones who get the most out of the courses, who make the biggest changes in their approach to life and who gain the greatest relief from their suffering. Sometimes the changes I witness seem miraculous.

When I met Derek he had been working in an operating theatre in a war zone. He held a senior role and we can only begin to imagine the horrors of what he saw daily, of the decisions he had to make. Now he was suffering from a combination of post-traumatic stress, insomnia, depression and agoraphobia – he could barely get out of the house. He wasn't sure any more whether life was worth living.

Despite all this, Derek managed to engage with the mindfulness practice and felt some real benefits. By practising mindfulness techniques such as the three-minute breathing space beforehand, he was gradually able to get out more. Then one day he spent five long minutes watching a beautiful butterfly. That butterfly helped him decide that life was wonderful, that it was worth living after all.

Derek was sufficiently motivated by the severity of his suffering to take responsibility for his healing, to sign up for the course, do the home practice and reap the benefits.

The power of beliefs

As life coach Fiona Harrold says, 'Beliefs have the potential to create or destroy . . . we come to accept them as absolute truths . . . choose to replace those that don't help and benefit you . . . choose beliefs that will open up possibilities and opportunities for you.'

This is crucial, especially whether we believe we can heal and go on to live a full and rewarding life or whether we believe we are stuck with a limiting psychiatric label for ever. One woman, Louise, who writes about her story in *From Recovery to Emancipation*, has this to say about the role and power of beliefs:

> It starts by . . . imagining and believing. Believing that you can work again, you can go out anywhere you choose, you can get in touch with those old friends, you can drive your car where you have never been before, you can make that telephone call and you can give your husband a cuddle without fearing it will lead to more!

She talks about taking a big gamble to come off medication:

> In terms of gambling on wellness and recovery, I started with a small stake and I won a little, but I liked winning, so I gambled again . . . I was confident that I was the one now that was in control and although I was always aware of the possibilities of losing, I now had the courage and determination to keep on taking those risks. I had belief that I could now be a winner and other people started to believe me.[13]

Crucially, she writes, 'I had to believe in myself when no one else did.' Finally she says, 'I sincerely hope that everyone has the chance and belief in themselves not to rely purely on traditional medical model interventions.'

Believing in herself and her ability to recover was of paramount importance. This underlines Fiona Harrold's assertion that beliefs have the power 'to create or destroy'. In this case, thanks to Louise's courage, they created a whole new life for her.

It might seem unusual quoting from a life coach when we're

exploring mental wellbeing. Life coaching is, however, now starting to be used specifically in the mental health field. This is an innovative and exciting development which I encourage you to explore if you feel drawn to it. As Louise says, 'With the right support you can achieve your goals.' The right support for you might well be a life coach with mental health expertise or a mental health practitioner using life-coaching skills.

We're going to look at this all-important issue of support in the next step, 'Reaching out'. We're ready now to start exploring the other steps, building on this first and fundamental one of taking responsibility. All the other steps become possible once we are ready to do this.

Step 2

Reaching out

'Validation is primary.'

Mary

With our seven steps, so far we've looked at taking responsibility for our healing. This particularly applies to the question of reaching out; we need to reach out to find support and validation, to find others who can help us. This is not necessarily easy, of course, and I know only too well what the challenges can be. The first is even knowing that we need help. If we have struggled alone for a long time, that can become a habitual pattern. It doesn't even occur to us this needs changing.

Many of us have been deeply scarred emotionally or psychologically and develop a fierce independence. This may have served us well as a coping mechanism for the intolerable situations we were in; now, however, we need to be realistic about when 'going it alone' isn't the best way.

The second challenge is being able to ask for help. In my experience, reaching out for support does gradually become easier, as we get to know ourselves better. We learn over time. We can help this process by initially asking for small things, things we feel comfortable asking for. Then we can move on to more challenging things. Along with asking, we can explain that we find it difficult to even ask.

Being validated

My story
In 2003 I had to travel back from a week in Egypt in a wheelchair. No broken bones – this was a result of the extreme psychospiritual crisis I had been through there. I had to take two months off work, but that was all. I didn't end up in hospital or on medication. Not only that, but I went on to make some very positive changes in my life. I left my job

and went on retreat for two months to give myself the time and space to fully integrate all I had been through. My whole life after that shifted direction. The outer changes, leaving my job and my flat, organizing a conference on spiritual crisis, merely reflected my inner transformation.

In that one week in Egypt I re-engaged with the natural process of healing and spiritual unfolding which had been so abruptly interrupted by my hospitalization years earlier, when I was 20. What was it that made such a difference? Why had I ended up in hospital the first time, losing a year of my life, yet this time was able to move through to such a positive outcome? One of the most important factors was simply that this time my experience was validated by people around me. My therapist and the training staff at the Karuna Institute were particularly supportive. They expected me not only to come through, but to come through better for this healing crisis. They didn't see it as 'illness', something 'wrong' with me, but as an opportunity. Their confidence gave me confidence, despite the terrifying place I had been to. And of course, thanks to that, I more than fulfilled their expectations for me.

This is what we mean by being validated, by having our experience validated. It can make the whole difference between those who flounder and those who flourish. In Chapter 5, on 'More healing approaches', we will hear about some individuals and projects that have achieved good results by keeping medication to a minimum. Lauren Mosher, John Weir Perry, Abram Hoffer, mental health services in west Lapland, all have one other thing in common: they expect their patients and clients to get better. They expect them to do well. They have seen just that, time and time again, and have no reason to doubt it. 'The message that we give is that we can manage this crisis. We have experience that people can get better, and we have trust in this kind of possibility,' say the Finnish therapists.

The vital importance of such a positive validating message cannot be overemphasized. It is crucial to our wellbeing at such a vulnerable time. It is crucial to the outcome. If a person in authority and power, such as a psychiatrist, tells us that our 'illness' is chronic, that we will have recurring episodes and need to take medication for the rest of our life, and if they tell us that when we are at our most vulnerable, many are likely to believe it. And we have already seen the power of beliefs. If we are not aware of evidence to the contrary, we are even more likely to believe such a dismal prognosis. Just being given the opposite, a validating message, is powerful enough to make all the difference. Below is Jane's story, which dramatically illustrates the contrast.

Spiritual emergence versus bipolar – a personal story

Three years ago I went through a spontaneous spiritual emergence. When I look back remembering that time, I can say that the day my crisis peaked was the most important day of my life. Although the experience was scary and disorientating at times, because I had no understanding of what was happening to me, it was transcendental and profound overall and I consider it to have been a healing gift. More than anything the experience was a chance to reset my life so that I was able to move forward free of the heavy emotional hurts I had been carrying.

The two years leading up to my crisis were the hardest of my life. I was trying to get my career started but met with rejection at every turn. However, as I reflect now, I consider the struggle I experienced leading up to my crisis to be a part of the wider spiritual emergence process itself. In my case it was as if I needed to be brought to my lowest point so that my ego finally surrendered to my heart. All the while I had been trying to get my first proper job following university, my head and heart had been in conflict – I insisted to myself I wanted a normal job, but I realize now that I would have hated working in an office, living a regular tick-tock life, which was what I was pushing and striving for at the time. It took me two years of struggle and closed doors followed by a big personal catastrophe to get me to finally listen to what my heart had been urging me to do all along – begin working for myself.

When things fell apart for me, it happened with a bang within the space of 24 hours. Relationships that had been constants in my life were suddenly gone: a long-term relationship I was in ended and also a family argument happened which caused separation and distance to occur between us. On top of this, I had to move house. However, when so much change happens as if out of nowhere, it makes it somewhat easier to carve out a new path for yourself. Importantly, I carved out my own path and chose to do exactly what felt right for me, against the advice of controlling family members.

The spiritual emergence process seems to work in terms of contrasts and symmetry. It was around four months after my collapse that the spiritual emergence process peaked for me. The day itself was somehow more alive from the start. I remember being in the shower and having the sensation that the water was washing away all the hurt and struggle I'd been going through for so long. By the end of my shower I felt light, free and full of buzzing energy.

My strange shower experience was followed by what I would

describe as a high-energy day full of energizing encounters and events seeming to be filled with deeper, symbolic significance. This day was also different in terms of the enhanced visual perception I experienced throughout – everything was brighter and looked somehow more real than usual.

It was at night time that things took a more frightening turn. My senses had sharpened to the point where I could smell food that was in the kitchen fridge, a long way from my bedroom. I felt I could also hear conversations that were happening in my neighbours' houses. This particularly worried me as my association with hearing noises was that it was a sign of schizophrenia. Were the voices I heard those of my neighbours? Or were they just voices in my head? There was nothing else for me to do except lie in bed with far too much energy to sleep while my powerful senses were working overload and frightening me.

While lying in bed I became disorientated as I listened to fragments of conversations taking place among people I didn't know. At some point I slipped into a trance state in which pulsations of electrical energy hummed their way up and down my body. I did not know what these sensations were but I was not afraid of them because they were more pleasurable than any bodily sensation I had ever experienced. Then, there was a 'pop' and suddenly my consciousness was no longer in my body. I could not see where I was but I experienced joining all things in oneness. I don't know how long I was outside my body because there was no sense of time in that place. This out-of-body experience and moment of metaphysical realization about all things being one formed the peak of my spiritual emergence.

My spiritual emergence was something I went through privately. I did not tell my family what had happened to me because I knew it was not something they would be able to understand. Since my closest relationships with friends and family had also broken down a couple of months previously, in a sense I also had enough distance from others to move through the process on my own. If anyone thought I was acting out of character at the time while my heightened state continued over the following weeks, nobody intervened, perhaps because there was no single person to have observed me on a daily basis.

Following the peak of my spiritual emergence, my energy stayed high for a couple of weeks, though importantly I was in control of the additional influx of energy throughout. During this time I was able to continue with my normal life and routines, albeit with an ecstatic glow surrounding me. While the energy stayed strong in me I began to wonder if I might have some kind of spiritual superpowers, since my own high energy appeared to influence the people and situations taking place around me. As the energy faded over the coming weeks, I let this idea go and steadily became more grounded.

In the months and years that followed my spiritual emergence, I came to understand that I was not alone in having gone through the process. There's even a possibility that it's actually a lot more widespread than is currently known. First, it's extremely hard to describe the process of spiritual emergence in language; it may be that many people may have been through something similar but they lack the language and concepts required to communicate their experience. Second, those who pass through the process may wish to keep quiet about it out of fear that other people won't understand and will label such experiences 'psychosis'.

I have seen in my own personal experience that the process of emergence is delicate and in some cases may be hijacked by the involvement or interference of the wrong people. It seems to me that there is a very fine line between experiencing a spiritual emergence and being labelled with having bipolar disorder.

My current boyfriend had his first manic episode when he was nineteen. When it happened he experienced his heart opening to feel love and connectedness to all people. The feeling lasted for three weeks, at which point he confided in his family. They were not at all understanding of what he was going through and his telling them about his experience of unconditional love ended with a stay in mental hospital, medications and being given the 'bipolar' label.

When I was originally told this story by my boyfriend, the similarity between our experiences struck me. In both cases our energy climbed to a high state which was maintained over a period of weeks. We also both experienced the same feeling of connection to all things. The major difference between us was that my experience was a private one, whereas in my boyfriend's case his controlling family had become involved and pursued the well-trodden path of labels and medications. In my boyfriend's situation things are further complicated by his Middle Eastern background. While I was able to ride through my process myself, for him there was no going back once his controlling family became involved.

My boyfriend has not been continuously taking medication since his first manic episode. Since I had only known him to be stable during our relationship, I doubted the official bipolar diagnosis. From the way he had described it to me, what he went through all those years before during his first manic episode seemed to be just another name for the same process I had myself experienced. To me the major difference between us was that he had put his trust in fearful people who did not understand the spiritual aspect of his experiences.

I later got to see my boyfriend having a manic episode at first hand. As I watched him go through the process there were many echoes to my own experience of crisis in terms of his altered perception and experience of time not being real. I remember thinking that if only I knew how to ground him it might be possible to stop things escalating further and preventing a full-blown manic episode. However, I was not able to stop him from wanting to go out and explore, and because of this I turned to his family for help, feeling by this point that I was out of my depth and had no other contacts. Within 24 hours his family had him sectioned again and during his three-week stay in hospital he was given a course of ECT (electro-convulsive therapy).

What I saw of my boyfriend's behaviour during the two days I was with him during his manic episode is that his expression of 'madness' was a form of healing of deep personal significance to him. For example, when his family arrived they did not come with love and compassion. They forced him to go with them as if he were a prisoner on his way to jail. During this time he was laughing and hugging them and at one point told everybody to start salsa dancing! While this may sound like crazy behaviour, in my opinion his behaviour is deeply symbolic in terms of his family and their issues. This is because his family are extremely serious people who do not laugh or smile. It seemed to me that only by going 'mad' in this way was he able to express how he really felt and how he wished to be seen within the family. It was as if he needed the crisis to be able to show them his playful and fun nature that is normally kept hidden from them because of their seriousness.

During two days of watching him go through his process I felt sure that I was watching a profound healing experience which was bringing up deeply buried hurts from his psyche. If only I had been able to keep him grounded and prevent his need to wander, perhaps then he could have had a successful spiritual emergence.

The situation now is that my boyfriend is out of hospital and is once again on a regime of bipolar medication. His family are extremely fearful of relapse and have full faith in doctors, ECT, medications and their injections. While I recognize that their concern is because they worry about him harming himself during a manic episode, their actions seem to be borne more out of their need to control him rather than being acts of loving care and emotional support. They do not believe healing is possible, because in their opinion 'bipolar' is an incurable disease. Plus, they are unwilling to listen to alternative viewpoints or accept the spiritual significance of mania.

While you can show someone the shadow of how a different future may be possible for them away from labels and medications, it is not possible for you to make that decision for somebody else because it involves taking full responsibility of your own life and letting go of relationships that are no longer serving you. It also means ignoring what doctors tell you and instead placing your faith in yourself and the unknown. I stand here now offering my support to my boyfriend, but I'm not sure he is ready to strike out for himself away from his family's control. More than this, it takes deep inner strength to earnestly want to heal by facing the wounds deep in one's psyche, and for many people it's too much to ask, since it's so much easier to pop a pill and do what the doctors tell you.

Based on what I have seen happens in his country's private mental health system, I have no faith that the system is designed around meeting patients' needs. It seems to work well for the hospitals who are making money from courses of ECT and lifetime prescriptions, but for individuals like my partner, whose experience of a manic episode is so similar to my own spiritual emergence, I feel in my heart there has to be a better path, which if pursued could over time lead to deep healing such as I myself have experienced.

As we can see from Jane's story, finding those who can and will validate our journey relates closely to the issue of support. At such times of crisis, support needs to come from those who are genuinely able to validate what we are going through. If family and friends are fearful and see us as 'ill', then we need to look elsewhere for support. In all our interactions, as we reach out for help we need to be aware of the individual's perspective. If we bear in mind the vital importance of being validated then we can avoid those who are not able to do this and seek out those who can.

Is your experience being validated?

- Does the person simply want to control and suppress symptoms?
- Is she using the pathologizing language of 'illness'?
- Does she think there is something 'wrong' with you?

Or . . .

- Does that person trust the process you are going through?
- Does she see it as an opportunity for real healing, for deep healing?
- Is she interested in what is going on beneath the surface?

Sources of support

Hopefully, much of our support will come from family and friends, those who love us and care about us. It is, however, a very good idea to reach out beyond family and close friends. This is partly because we need other kinds of support too, such as professional health expertise. It is also because the wider network of support we have, the better.

Our wider community

An example of an extraordinary network of spiritual support for those struggling with any kind of issue relating to addiction (not necessarily your own) is the worldwide Alcoholics Anonymous (AA) fellowship, encompassing Narcotics Anonymous, Codependants Anonymous, Adult Children of Alcoholics and more.

With the internet, our wider community has also gained a global dimension. Online support groups and networks tend to be issue-focused, such as the UK Spiritual Crisis Network, which offers email contact for those struggling with psychospiritual issues. (The equivalent in Canada is the Spiritual Emergence Service which has a free telephone helpline.) There are also support groups, such as the mental health charity Sane's online forum, as well as many communities focusing on, for instance, bipolar or depression. A very large online community in the United States is madinamerica.com. If you want to find out about online safety guidelines, the charity Mind has a useful guide, 'How to stay safe online', on its website. All the details mentioned in this paragraph and elsewhere in the book are listed in the Useful addresses section.

One issue to be aware of is our tendency, with any one community, to get stuck in a certain identity: I am 'this' or I am 'that'. We want to be changing and growing, and perceiving ourselves with a fixed label can hold us in a stuck place. As we change and grow, clinging to a set identity or illness label does not do justice to our progress along the healing path. That said, such communities can be a wonderful help when we most need it, as long as we recognize when it's time to move on.

Be aware also that information shared on those online forums can be word of mouth and anecdotal. It may not be totally reliable. You need to always check against sources you consider to be reliable. If I want to try a particular natural remedy, say, for helping to have less restless sleep, I use my own version of triangulation, a research method for checking results. If I find the same positive information from three independent and reliable sources then I consider it to be good. On the same basis, information about a particular psychiatric drug from the manufacturer who produced it is not sufficiently independent.

The recovery community

The mental health recovery community deserves a special mention, given its potential relevance to your healing journey. Coming out of the influential work of Mary Ellen Copeland in the USA, her WRAP (Wellness Recovery Action Plan) and training has been very popular and widely taken up. It has given rise to an entire recovery movement. I've avoided using the term 'recovery' on the whole, however, because I find it can be confusing. Many use it to refer to 'managing illness' or 'managing symptoms'. For me, real healing, recovery in its deepest and fullest sense, means living without symptoms, living a full and rich life, in the way that people like Cathy Penney, who wrote the Foreword, do.

The voluntary and charity sector

Within mental health, there is a vast array of groups, projects and organizations at both national and local level. Self-injury Support, which specializes in supporting women and girls who self-harm, has a national remit. Mind and Rethink, the mental health charities, have local groups in many towns, though often with little or no emphasis on the transpersonal or spiritual dimension. However, these kinds of organizations tend to offer free or low-cost support, which can be crucial at such times.

The important advantage of online communities, the recovery community and the voluntary and charity sectors is that the support available is usually peer support; it is from people who have been through something similar. If you have not experienced this before it is difficult to convey in words how supportive that can feel.

Health professionals

The right healthcare professional, or professionals, for you can also be incredibly supportive. In Step 3 we'll look in detail at how to get the support you need from health professionals, whether mainstream or integrative.

Step 3

Finding the right healthcare professional

'Trust your gut.'

Marie

My story

The psychiatrist who declared that 'sometimes it's best not to try to understand these things' was clearly not the right healthcare professional for me. Years later, when I was referred to a psychologist for cognitive behavioural therapy (CBT), this started to feel more in line with my needs. It came at a time when I was learning to meditate. The psychologist was as fascinated as I was in the cross-over between the mindfulness principles in CBT and my meditation. At the same time I had asked to be referred for psychotherapy on the NHS. I had an initial assessment appointment, but the waiting list was so long that by the time an appointment actually came through I had moved away from the area.

While I was waiting I asked around and found a private Gestalt therapist, on personal recommendation from a trusted colleague. I worked with her for six months. So, although the CBT was a step in the right direction, it was really only when I started to look beyond the NHS that I began to find the help I needed. As I came to see my journey as one of healing and growth the NHS model of care felt less and less appropriate for me.

I also started doing group therapeutic work on a course at the Karuna Institute. As I embarked on their first year of psychotherapy training I started working with a therapist experienced in their Core Process psychotherapy approach. I continued working with that therapist for several years and it was a truly transformative experience for me. I was healing emotionally and psychologically, gaining an inner strength and resilience. He had complete faith in my ability to move successfully through periods of crisis and, as you would expect from a good therapist, he supported me totally and unconditionally.

What issue do you need help with?

Some 50 per cent of those in psychiatric hospital have suffered some form of abuse, physical or sexual. This does not include all those who have been emotionally abused and all those who are not even aware that they have been abused, that what they have been subjected to was abusive. For instance, I had no idea until much later in life that my father's behaviour was verbally and emotionally damaging. I used to end up in abusive relationships without even realizing that a boyfriend's behaviour was unacceptable. You don't have to have been physically hit to have suffered traumatic abuse.

You also don't have to have been physically hit to access services from domestic violence projects. Domestic violence, where intimidation is used systematically to control a partner, can be emotional, psychological, financial or sexual, not only physical. The same goes for sexual abuse. There is a whole range of trauma, which goes from being touched inappropriately as a child to non-consensual sex between husband and wife.

Both domestic violence and sexual abuse services offer free support. If you have been physically or sexually abused, either in the past or more recently, a specialist agency may have the right kind of expertise for you. Reaching out for this kind of help could well be an important part of your healing journey. I appreciate that just picking up the phone or sending an email to make that first contact may not be easy. If so, ask somebody you trust to help you take that first step.

Looking for an expert, someone with specialist expertise, is generally a very good idea. Whether you're struggling, for instance, with depression, with voices or with some form of trauma, you can look for someone who specializes in that and who has a track record of helping others to heal. When I use the word 'heal' I don't mean simply controlling symptoms. Don't settle for that. You deserve so much more.

Which therapeutic approach?

In looking for the right healthcare professional, you need to decide which path you want to go down. Which therapeutic approach resonates with you? As Dr Andrew Powell, the psychiatrist and therapist, rightly points out, the spiritual or soul-centred approach is not for everyone. 'Many human problems can be explored and resolved psychodynamically . . . [some] patients simply prefer to stay firmly grounded in the affairs of daily life.' If this is the case for you, there is plenty of choice, from a whole range of talking therapies to nutritional therapy, mindfulness, life coaching, home-opathy and more. You need to think about whether you want to take a more orthodox approach or look for holistic practitioners, or even a combination of both. Increasingly we are seeing this combined, integrated approach, such as where shiatsu or yoga are available on psychiatric wards.

There are also more and more professionals trained in both con-ventional and natural medicine. This can be very helpful.

During the early stages of your healing journey, which are often the most intense, you may benefit from more than one approach, more than one professional, or even a whole team. This could also be the case if your specific needs require a particular specialism. For instance, you might be under the care of a psychiatrist and also see a nutritionist and/or psychotherapist. The important thing is to keep everybody informed.

> One of my mindfulness students came to me at the end of an eight-week course. Thanks to what he had gained from the course, he was now keen to come off anti-depressant medication and felt ready to do so. Please note, this is not something I ever suggest or recommend. It has to be entirely the individual's choice and decision. What I did recom-mend was that he seek one-to-one support while doing that, such as counselling or psychotherapy. Anti-depressants suppress emotions, so as we start to come off them the original emotional and psychological pain may rise to the surface again, needing to be addressed. I felt my student needed support to be able to deal with this healing process.

How do you find the right health professional?

Everybody's healing journey is unique. No two will be the same. Given my particular path, I have a personal bias towards what has worked for me, in particular transpersonal psychotherapy, mindful-ness and Deep Memory Process therapy. When you're looking for certain health professionals, such as therapists, it can be helpful to have met them in another context and got a sense of them as a person: for example, hearing them speak at a conference or attending a workshop led by them. If there is someone you're interested in, find out what events that person may have coming up that you could go to. The therapist I worked with for several years was one of the trainers on my psychotherapy course, so I had a good sense of him when I chose him.

When I hear of people who have tried talking therapy but didn't find it of much use, I wonder whether this is because they have not found a good, professional therapist, who is right for them. These three criteria, of whether someone is professional in his practice, good at what he does and right for you, are important whatever kind of health practitioner you are looking for. Some therapists will offer a free first meeting, which is not an actual session. This is an opportunity to find out as much about them as you can. Don't be afraid to ask any of the questions below.

The two main professional bodies in the UK for counsellors and psychotherapists are the British Association for Counselling and Psychotherapy (BACP) and the UK Council for Psychotherapy (UKCP). Through their online directories you can search by geographical area and also by therapeutic approach, such as transpersonal, person-centred or Jungian.

Is the practitioner professional?

- What are her qualifications?
- What training has she had?
- How long was it?
- How long has she been practising?
- If relevant, what supervision does she have?
- Is she registered with a recognized association?
- If so, does it have a code of practice and a complaints procedure?
- Are these publicly available?
- Is she covered by professional indemnity insurance?
- Will your records be confidential?
- How does she view any orthodox medication or health care you may be having?
- Is she professional in the way she presents and conducts herself?

These questions are adapted from Dr Jan Wallcraft's *Healing Minds* report, published by the Mental Health Foundation.

If you're looking for low-cost therapeutic support from a counsellor or psychotherapist, bear in mind that students tend to charge much lower rates. The added advantage is that, because they are trainees, they will be receiving much more supervision and guidance than would normally be the case. Students who are not yet fully qualified will not be listed in the BACP or UKCP directories. You will need to approach training schools, such as the Karuna Institute, Re-Vision or the Centre for Counselling and Psychotherapy Education, directly (see the Useful addresses section).

Is the practitioner good at what he or she does?

Personal recommendation from someone whose opinion you trust can be very helpful here. Another guide is that he or she may have a reputation locally for being good. As Dr Jan Wallcraft writes in the *Healing Minds* report, 'Be wary of anyone who claims to perform "miracles" or promises to cure you.' She also recommends keeping a log of your wellbeing during treatment to gauge what progress you feel you are making. If you're not happy, discuss it with the practitioner, then consider finding someone else. Be aware, however, that with talking therapy it can be tempting to give up when the going gets a bit tough, which, if it's working, it invariably will.

Is the practitioner right for you?

- Do you feel comfortable with the practitioner?
- Do you like him or her?
- Is he or she willing to truly listen to what you have to say?
- Do you feel heard?
- Do you feel your thoughts, feelings, wishes are being respected?

Here are Marie's thoughts on finding the right person:

> In the UK one of the ways to find a potential therapist is to look up the Counselling Directory online. All the therapists registered have met requirements and you can look at their photos and descriptions of their work and find out who is in your area. Then trust your gut. For me this means listening closely to my own experience and feeling of ease around someone as a priority over what qualifications he or she may have. What do I experience when I'm with the practitioner? Am I censoring what I share – and if I don't, what do I notice in his response? Does he allow me to work at my own pace? Is he able to slow things

down and give me space to explore what arises? Do I feel liked? Do I leave the appointment standing on my own two feet, even during difficult times?

Like Catherine, I absorbed what it was to grow up with an abusive parent. One of the effects of this was to be often unaware of my choices and live with behaviour from others that was in reality unacceptable to me. When crisis hit 20 years ago, I was lucky enough to be recommended an Alexander Technique practitioner by a friend, a very gentle man who seemed gifted in providing the sort of listening and attention to the body that I needed.

I discovered from this that I am personally drawn to therapies that explicitly include the body as first point of contact. It seems natural to trust my own real experience in the here and now and learn to re-inhabit my own skin, something which was hard to do in the early days. Over the years the positive results of this process have led me to explore working within the models of psychosynthesis, Gestalt, focusing, tantra, yoga and dance movement psychotherapy, where I currently feel most at home.

Changing professional

We need professionals who believe in our ability to heal, rather than simply managing symptoms for the rest of our lives. Linking in with the previous step, we need to assess whether or not our key healthcare professional is validating our recovery. Does he or she believe in our capacity to heal? Here are the kind of questions to be considering again:

How to gauge whether your experience is being validated

- Does the person trust the process you are going through?
- Does he or she see it as an opportunity for real healing, for deep healing?
- Is he or she interested in what is going on beneath the surface?

Or . . .

- Does the practitioner simply want to control and suppress symptoms?
- Is he or she using the pathologizing language of 'illness'?
- Does he or she think there is something 'wrong' with you?

If your practitioner does not believe in your ability to heal, then you need to go elsewhere. This is about not giving our power away. While health professionals may be experts in their field, we are the expert on ourselves. If our practitioner is not validating our recovery then we need to change and find someone else who will. This is subtly different from Wallcraft's caution to be wary of those who promise to cure you. You are the one doing the growing, changing and healing, and while professionals can support you in this, nobody can do it for you, nobody can cure you. As Dr Powell puts it: 'our patients already hold the key to their own healing, if only helped to make use of it'.

If, for example, you decide you want to gradually come off medication, you will need to be very clear about whether your doctor or psychiatrist believes in your ability to heal. You need medical support as you slowly taper off, and if he or she does not know or trust that healing is possible, you will need to find someone who does. Explore this fully with your practitioner, with the help of an advocate if need be. It may be a question of having more than one professional in place towards the beginning, when you need most help. Would they be willing to back you if you had plenty of support in place, such as one-to-one therapy?

Remember that many psychiatrists, through no fault of their own, have sadly been trained to believe that therapy can aggravate certain states. This is not surprising, especially in the United States, where Dr Bertram Karon tells us that virtually all postgraduate education in psychiatry today is paid for by drug companies. There is plenty of evidence that most people who get real therapy do heal, including the work of Dr Daniel Dorman, Dr Bertram Karon, Dr Jean Marc Mantel and many more.

Changing health professional is easier in countries like the United States, where the medical system is set up completely differently from the UK's NHS. However, in the UK you can go back to your GP and ask to be referred to a different psychiatrist.

In the next step, we turn to those who have turned their lives around. We will see how these individuals have followed the 'Seven steps to healing', how they have taken responsibility for their wellbeing, reached out for support, found those who validate their journey, and put the right health care in place.

Step 4

Focusing on success stories

'Our unbreakable inner self is waiting to be found.'

Ursula

Think of the 'Seven steps to healing' as strategies for success. It makes sense, then, to focus on stories of success. We need to find out how others have gone about it. What worked for them? Reading or hearing about other people's success can be inspiring, uplifting and encouraging – hugely so.

This is partly why Alcoholics Anonymous and other 12-step pro- grammes work so well. Every meeting involves someone sharing his or her story. Those further ahead on their journey of recovery share their stories with newcomers. So when you're asking around among family and friends or surfing the online communities, looking for people who have struggled with similar experiences, look for those who are now doing really well. Look for those who are further ahead on their healing journey than you. What worked for them? See if any of it resonates with you.

Part of the difficulty for psychiatrists, again through no fault of their own, is that they rarely get to see the success stories. How many of us, once we've turned our lives around, actually go back to show them what can be done? Very few of us, I suspect. So it's all too easy for psychiatrists to believe their own dire prognoses, that many mental health 'illnesses' are for life and that patients will have to take medication for the duration of that life.

Meet Ursula and Hamilton. They share their stories here in their own words. Both raise issues that touch on the complex relation- ship between mysticism and mental health, between breakdown and breakthrough. For a full discussion of these issues you can read my book *In Case of Spiritual Emergency*.

Ursula has been admitted to psychiatric wards in England, France and New Zealand, ten times in all. Twice she was sec- tioned, held under the Mental Health Act. A high-flying young public relations consultant in London when her first crisis struck, she found herself on a rollercoaster journey that stripped her of everything she knew – career, relationships, friends. Psychospiritual crisis or spiritual emergency can do this sometimes, bringing about profound personal transformation. Difficult as it may be to believe, few, if any, have any regrets about the direction their life takes.

Today, Ursula's hard-won inner peace and contentment come hand in hand with a loving husband and a little girl. Her story of success speaks volumes about the first of our seven steps, taking responsibility for our own healing.

The unbreakable place

I believe that our unbreakable inner self is waiting to be found, like a long-lost loved one. It animates us at our fundamental level of pure being, before instinct, thought or emotion. I went looking for it in 1997. I found it and, although it broke me, I touched the face of God. Now I have the arms of that long-lost loved one wrapped around me and we have melted into an everyday wholeness. This is my story of how I have survived spiritual emergence.

My first emergence in January 1998 led me into psychiatric hospital. For over a year I had been pursuing a spiritual path. I read New Age books and started following any signs of synchronicity. I started having acupuncture, I had a past-life reading, I started meditation and yoga. I studied hands-on healing. I became vegetarian and consciously energized and cleansed my food. I went on a spiritual retreat over New Year and a couple of weeks later I had my first experience of a psychotic thought, or a spiritual emergence manifestation. I was convinced I was pregnant by immaculate conception. That was a Friday. By Sunday, events had escalated on a truly epic scale and I was the living embodiment of the Goddess, having married the Christ and also been overshadowed by the Virgin Mary on the Saturday. I could no longer answer to my given earthly name.

I believe it is possible that if that first experience had been handled very differently, I may not have had as many further hospital admissions. I have had ten in total. I do feel that I have needed the safety of a secure place when each of my episodes or emergences has manifested, and while I have at times rebelled against and baulked at the established psychiatric model which has held me in place, it has held me in place and saved my life. There was never any other option available to me. I can put my hand on my heart and say that despite enforced injections, the whirlwind of anti-psychotic medication and the daily dose I still take,

I am no poorer spiritually for it. The little pills with big names pack a powerful pathological punch but they cannot ever touch or tarnish my unbreakable self. I am now perfectly content to work with psychiatric medication. I find that it provides my body with the support it needs. Changing my attitude towards medication has been a fundamental key to freeing me from some very limiting thought patterns.

If I look scrupulously carefully at what has effectively brought about my survival through 16 years of pure spiritual crisis and battle with my bipolar diagnosis, it is one thing: my attitude. Nothing else. I have had to take full responsibility for my thoughts, feelings and opinions. When I was trying to see everything from a purely spiritual perspective and feeling persecuted by the psychiatric mainstream, I tied myself in knots searching for all the answers alone. When I lost faith and turned my back on my inner world and followed mainstream medicine to the letter, I felt stifled and choked, as if chains were being wound around me. After oscillating between these polar points of view, I found the middle way. For me, the balance I needed was born in my mind when I realized that *I am all I have*. I must therefore be responsible for identifying and sourcing what I need to function, thrive and find joy in life. It sounds obvious, but this was a massive turning point because I always searched for all the answers from outside sources – books, therapists, yoga, meditation, spiritual teachers, prayer, reiki, psychiatrists, acupuncture, flower essences, more books, angels, crystals, tarot, more therapists and every New Age course that 'resonated' with me. I have always had a tendency to try to award expert or guru-like status to someone in a position of power in the desperate hope that the proverbial light bulb would come on in their presence. But they always had feet of clay and something always shattered the bulb before I discovered enough anyway.

The light bulb moment came to me on my own. I woke up into a full realization about myself and the nature of my wholeness. I saw how the spiritual and psychiatric worlds each hold a unique set of complementary keys both vital to me. For example, my spiritual path and practices have honed my instincts and sensitivities to such a fine tuning that I trust them with regard to the choices I make about my care from the mainstream psychiatric model. I choose to remain on daily medication and follow my instincts with consultative reassessment where necessary. I do not feel spiritually duller or dumbed down, where I once did many years ago while on medication. Nor do I preach spiritual perspective upon the ears of mainstream medical men and women as I once felt compelled to do. It feels far more honest now simply to witness and observe the inescapably spiritual nature of any person or situation. Having been a bit evangelical about the wonders of the New Age as I discovered them many years ago, now I love the silence.

I would love to present myself as some sort of Tolkien elf – graciously in this world and yet not of it. But the wonderful human truth is that I am very much of this world. I have real, deep, living trauma and plenty of demons to keep me awake at night. But the opposite is true too. I have flown with angels and have found a precious living balance filled with very great joy indeed. I would be lying if I said I didn't wish there were some things I could change. But this entire experience has broken me open. And that is how I found what I was looking for.

Ursula's powerful story illustrates how our awakening can tip over into crisis. She accurately points to the crucial importance of how our first 'break' is handled, something the Open Dialogue therapists we will hear about in Chapter 4 seem to understand. As we open up to and tap into the energy of the Divine it is not uncommon to experience the energy of the Christ consciousness or the Virgin Mary.

Hamilton shares next. In terms of our seven steps, his story highlights how helpful it was for him when he found the right healthcare professionals, when he got rid of the toxic, in his case alcohol, and when he reached out for support from those who were able to validate his experience.

Psychedelics to psychosis: the journey of a spiritual seeker

A search for a deeper connection – a spiritual dimension – started in my late teens. In those days the vehicle of choice was psychedelics. The few LSD trips I took exposed me to unbelievable realms, to a degree that my view of so-called 'reality' was changed for ever. This was sometimes an uncomfortable coexistence with the 'real' world so, many years later, my quest for meaning took me to India.

My first journey found me in Trivandrum, in southern India, participating in a two-week 'yoga vacation camp' in the Sivananda Ashram. This consisted of an austere programme where we got up at dawn and practised yoga meditation, asanas (body exercises), breathing practice and teaching from various yogic masters, until I fell into bed exhausted. This was for me a strict discipline, but when I left I was floating in a cloud of bliss.

This short introduction whetted my appetite, so two years later I joined ten other Canadians on a three-week retreat into the heart of Mount Arunachala, also in southern India and a holy centre for many a spiritual seeker. This is when I experienced being rocketed into another dimension at the culmination of a six-hour puja (an Indian spiritual ceremony) led by an Indian Realized Master, or mystic, and for two weeks afterwards I was in the world, but not of it. The only way I can describe this experience was as being given a blast of cosmic energy.

When I returned to the West, I sank into a state of despair and depression, a diagnosis of bipolar disorder and the beginning of a decade of medication. I was mentally stable, but with an unquenchable thirst for connection to a life of the spirit.

Years later I was back in India as the assistant to a Kriya yoga teacher. This involved two hours of daily practice which resulted in unleashing an intense flow of energy, like an express train, up through my spine and into my head, my body convulsing uncontrollably. It left me in a world where thoughts no longer existed, suspended in a kind of blissful twilight zone where nothing else much mattered. Unfortunately I had to return to Canada soon after these experiences, and I plummeted into a state of hopeless despair where suicide seemed a very attractive option.

Fortunately I found an amazing healer, a compassionate psychiatrist, who determined that I was suffering from PTSD (post-traumatic stress disorder), due to unresolved traumatic events in my earlier life. His treatment, EMDR (Eye Movement Desensitization and Reprocessing), lifted me out of my depression. His opinion was that virtually all 'mental disorders', at their foundation, are caused by some kind of trauma. He also prescribed an anti-psychotic medication. I was never sure whether it was his treatment (which was incredibly liberating) or the medication that resulted in a period of mental stability. Perhaps it was a combination of both.

About a year later I decided on a complete life change: I was weary of the persona that I had carefully constructed over the years, along with all the expectations of others as to who I was, what I did, habits, behaviours: the whole package known as Hamilton. In essence, I pulled the rug from under this comfortable stasis, a deliberate destabilization. Most of my friends thought I was crazy, and that is what I became. The result was an impossibly explosive, uncontainable energy, akin to something bottled up inside like a pressure-cooker but unable to be expressed. I was caught in a kind of limbo but in constant anxiety, mental anguish, unable to sleep, combined with compulsive restlessness. In and out of hospital, fed on a diet of tranquillizers, I experienced a continued burning sensation located in the top of my head. I was so worried that I might have a brain tumour that I had a thorough brain scan that found no apparent explanation. A good friend had been a disciple of the same Indian mystic at whose feet I had my first cosmic blast. His explanation was that I was so open that I was literally taking on vast amounts of external energy through my crown which my body was unable to contain. His diagnosis fitted with similar spiritual transformations and beautifully explained the how and the why of my frightening experience, but offered no immediate 'fix'.

Thus the only apparent remedy was the psychiatric ward. Mercifully my experience was positive; I was lucky to have the best that the Canadian health system had to offer. My caretakers were incredibly compassionate and it was a Godsend to relieve my long-suffering wife, who had been my sole caretaker up to that point. I was discharged with a cocktail of four different medications, a pharmaceutical mix of anti-psychotics, anti-depressants and anti-anxiety meds. My daily diet consisted of a careful regimen of these various pills – but at least I wasn't in a constant state of distress. My free fall into hell had been arrested. I was dopey but somewhat sane.

The real remedy to my chaotic state was discovering a supportive community of like-minded souls, people who had undergone similar transformative experiences to mine. Like me, they had been diagnosed with a variety of mental disorders, had gone through the mental health system and had what is now termed 'lived experience'. I had finally found 'my tribe'. A group of us meet weekly as part of a local (Vancouver) Spiritual Emergence network. We discuss our daily challenges of integrating our altered states with 'normal existence' in a world that rarely acknowledges our experiences.

The underlying theme of my 'awakening' has been my participation in Alcoholics Anonymous. Despite sometimes being seen as a group for the losers in life, it is a profoundly spiritual programme that for 15 years has provided me regular spiritual nourishment. After a disastrous dissolution of my first marriage, alcohol became my regular medication of choice. I knew this path would lead me to ruin, so now I can tap into a fellowship that is available just about anywhere in the world, people who encourage me to go further and deeper daily, and understand the struggles we humans have with the expression of Spirit.

In addition I have a team of professional specialists readily available, if I wish to avail myself of the conventional 'medical model' of mental health. I am gradually weaning myself off the medications which have the worst side effects, so I can continue my journey of self-exploration.

Ursula's and Hamilton's stories are inspiring. They are stories of courage, determination and perseverance. The healing journey is not an easy one, yet as we tackle our wounding and trauma head on, we give ourselves the greatest possible gift, that of wholeness and happiness. We deserve nothing less.

Whenever you're feeling discouraged or disheartened come back to this chapter, to this particular step to healing: focusing on success stories. Think of Cathy Penney, in hospital for years on end and described as catatonic in her medical notes. Then watch her on YouTube in Daniel Mackler's film *Take These Broken Wings*, full of health, energy and vitality. Read her full story in Dr Daniel Dorman's extraordinary book *Dante's Cure*. Look for other testimonials on YouTube, find a TED Talk, read a personal account of a fellow traveller coming through to the other side, like Katie Mottram's *Mend the Gap*. Find those who struggled with similar issues and are now living full and rich lives. What worked for them can work for you. If their success is possible, so is yours.

Step 5

Doing away with the toxic

'I was able to move forward free from heavy emotional hurts I was carrying.'

Jane

When it comes to anything toxic, you have to be ruthless, drastic, even draconian. It all has to go! On whatever level, get rid of it, do away with it, eliminate it. Now! Or as soon as is practically possible.

We can't expect to heal or grow if we carry on doing things as we've always done them. Something needs to change. Our crisis is a very clear indication of that. Our psyche is literally crying out for some imbalance to be tended.

How much do we want to heal? How far are we prepared to go in order to heal? Are we willing to make whatever changes are necessary or are we maybe unconsciously limiting ourselves in some way? We come back now to the key questions we looked at in Step 1. If you sense any resistance, explore it with kindness and gentleness towards yourself. What's it about? What's underlying it? You can also go back and review Step 1. At this stage it can be very useful to work with a good life coach to help you put in place the changes you want to make.

So what needs to change? Two types of change are needed. One involves eliminating things which are maybe toxic in some way, things which are not helping. The other is about putting in place that which will help or nourish us, which we'll look at in Step 6, 'Making life changes'.

Doing away with the unhelpful

Getting rid of anything toxic to our mental health potentially covers every aspect of our lives.

My story

Over the years I've had to leave toxic work situations and toxic relationships. I've had to address ways of thinking, emotional and psychological habits, that were not supporting me. I've had to eliminate certain foods and drink from my diet. This may all sound rather negative, but for everything I've taken out of my life I've put something far, far more nourishing, supportive and loving in its place. My current life is virtually unrecognizable from how it used to be. I didn't achieve this level of change overnight, however. It's taken me 20 years or more to learn what is and isn't healthy for me, to learn to distinguish between the two, and the process is ongoing, always being refined.

In some cases, the deeper the wounding, the longer it can take to make all the changes we need in our lives. This isn't necessarily the case, though, and I certainly wouldn't want to put any limits on how rapidly you can create healthy transformation in your life. We are all unique. What works for one person isn't automatically right for another. The process is one of getting to know ourselves, of discovering what is damaging and what is nurturing to us personally.

Toxic emotions

Here is Katie Mottram's experience of working through and letting go of guilt, taken from her memoir *Mend the Gap*. Having realized the extent to which deep-seated feelings of guilt were holding her back, here she is having a therapy session to uncover their roots.

I had always been aware that I was carrying guilt about causing my mum's post-natal depression through being born, and guilt at destroying my marriage through not realising I was gay. But I thought that I had let that go now as I knew that I didn't need to reprimand myself for hurt I hadn't intended to cause. But I was about to discover that I was holding onto something, of which I had been completely unaware. 'Where are you?' Chris asked as she directed me to travel back to where my emotions were keeping me 'stuck'. 'I'm standing on an icy road,' I replied, the words leaving my mouth only then making me aware that I was back at the scene of my miscarriage 'and I can see my car crumpled against the tree.' 'And what are you feeling?' 'I'm relieved. Oh my God, I feel guilty because I'm relieved about losing my baby!' Chris gradually brought me back into the present moment as tears streamed down my cheeks. 'I had no idea,' I stated, shocked at the information I had just discovered. I had always thought that the guilt I felt was due to being responsible for causing the miscarriage. 'It's okay,' Chris reassured.[14]

Stress

Stress is considered a major factor in mental health issues. We're unlikely to be able to eliminate stress completely from our lives, but we can certainly reduce it considerably by learning which situations, and which people, we find stressful and learning a stress management tool such as mindfulness.

> One of my mindfulness students, Rachel, worked with young female offenders. She was suffering badly from stress, having to regularly deal with aggression at work, with clients or clients' parents being verbally abusive and physically threatening towards her. Stress is one thing, but she was also a 'class A' diabetic; stress could prove literally fatal as it affects the body's ability to take up insulin. Her very life depended on being able to regulate her insulin levels.
>
> One woman, a client's mother, had been threatening to beat Rachel up and seemed quite capable of it. She was particularly irate on the phone one day after her daughter had spent the night in a cell as a result of failing to turn up in court. After putting down the phone, Rachel reported the incident to the police. Asked if she wanted to press charges, she declined, although she said in the past she might well have done. She then did a three-minute breathing space, one of the mindfulness exercises I teach, and got on with her day. Meanwhile her colleagues were ranting and raving; would or wouldn't the woman carry out her threat? Rachel's insulin readings? They were doing fine.

Rachel was highly committed to doing the mindfulness home practice. She was soon rewarded with life-changing results. By learning mindfulness she was able to learn to deal effectively with the toxic effects of stress.

Another source of stress we may not be aware of is all the negative, depressing or downright traumatic news we are bombarded with daily. Try an interesting experiment: a 'news fast'. Dr Andrew Weil, author of *Spontaneous Healing*, suggests not watching the news on television, listening to it on the radio or reading it in a newspaper for a day, gradually building up, over a few weeks, to a whole week. At the end of that week, see how you feel. You may well find that you want to limit how much mainstream news you subject yourself to each day. A wonderful alternative is *Positive News*, a newspaper which comes out quarterly. It is inspiring and uplifting and gives a healthy perspective on world events. Former news presenter and journalist Martyn Lewis wholeheartedly supports *Positive News* and has spoken out against the unbalanced media coverage we routinely get.

Relationships: from pain to peace

Do you find the whole subject of relationships tricky? Many of us who carry early wounding do. I've certainly had my fair share of pain and misery on that front, which thankfully is all behind me now. Ursula and Hamilton, whom you met in the previous step, are testament that loving and lasting relationships are possible. For that to happen we need to be able to recognize relationships that are toxic in some way *and* we need to be able to walk away from them if and when we consider them beyond repair.

Some find it much more difficult to leave unhealthy relationships than others. Deep down, in the bottom of our heart, we may know we need to end it but can't quite bring ourselves to. If this is you, then find a way of getting the support you need in order to be able to leave. If need be, seek professional counselling or psychotherapy to help you. Other times we may not even realize that the relationship we're in is abusive in some way. Emotional and psychological abuse can be very subtle. We may be very accustomed to behaviour that others wouldn't find acceptable. If our self-esteem is low owing to childhood wounding, on some level we may not feel we deserve any better. Again, we may need professional help.

The permutations of relationship situations are endless. Ask yourself a fundamental question: is this relationship making me happy? Is it supporting my mental health? Or not? Remember that our healing must take precedence over all else. Once our health and life are back on track, then we can create or attract healthier, more loving relationships.

Relationships are, of course, not limited to a significant other but extend to our wider families, friends and work colleagues. A situation at work where we are not being valued or treated appropriately, with respect and consideration, can bring untold misery and certainly needs addressing. Again, it may be that the way forward is to seek professional help, especially if the problem feels particularly intractable. You could do this through your trade union, if you have one. When it comes to work and career, seeing a life coach can also be very helpful, especially if we need to leave a job but can't see a way forward or any other options. Again, ask yourself: is this work situation supporting my mental health or not? What needs to change for it to do so?

House or home?

Just as who we live with can have a huge impact on our wellbeing, so too can where we live and how we live. Here is a clue: do you love where you're living?

My story
Three years after my husband and I split up I was still living in the home we had lived in together. I got back from a week's retreat and it suddenly dawned on me that, as lovely as the house was, I needed to move on. To move on with my life, I needed to move on to a new home.

Sometimes we don't need to actually move. We just need to clear out old energy, energy that may be stale and stagnant and keeping us stuck. Spring cleaning or decorating will help, but nothing beats a good old clear-out. I'm a firm believer in the power of clutter clearing as a way of shifting energy and shifting our lives. If you have never tried this, I highly recommend as a starting point Karen Kingston's excellent little book *Clear Your Clutter with Feng Shui*. Although she refers to feng shui at times, you don't need to have an interest in this in order to get a huge amount out of her book. Clutter clearing is a powerful way of creating change, of getting rid of the toxic. It's fantastically liberating and, what's more, it's fun.

Detoxing

When it comes to our health, clutter clearing also works wonders for our bodies. Detoxing is a powerful way of creating change and can dramatically impact on our mental health. From avoiding the likes of dairy products, meat, sugar, tea, coffee and alcohol for a week or two, to using herbs to help cleanse the colon, to juicing and fasting, there are many degrees of detoxing. And if you have old emotional baggage you want to clear out and move on from, nothing beats colonic irrigation. We all need to take good care of our colons. Just as we spring clean our homes, so a spring clean for our bodies after winter is a very good idea.

Diet

If we want to eliminate toxicity from our bodies, diet is important. This is especially so if you are taking or have taken medication which invariably has toxic side effects. The link between diet and mental health is now indisputable. There is so much research showing we can take better care of ourselves through our diet. Sensitivity to gluten, dairy or soya is very common. Nutritionists have found that eliminating one or more of these from the diet can make a vast difference to some people's mental wellbeing. Many of us 'sensitives' experience these items as toxic to our bodies. Try eliminating one of these at a time for two to four weeks and see what difference you notice.

Many people now appreciate the need to avoid stimulants such as tea, coffee and alcohol, although they don't necessarily find it easy to do. We often use these, as well as 'comfort' food, to suppress emotions. Alcohol is a depressant, so is particularly bad news if you're struggling with depression. Sugar and sweet food, including all the hidden sugar in our diets, are also highly addictive. They create spikes in blood sugar levels which anybody with mental health issues needs to avoid. If cutting these things out feels too much, then look for delicious, healthy alternatives, so that you feel you're having a treat rather than missing out. Try substituting fruit for cakes, for instance – but not any old fruit, your absolute favourite! Fizzy drinks tend to have aspartame as a sweetener. Aspartame is highly controversial and was banned for many years in the United States. Be particularly wary of anything that claims to be sugar-free.

Chronic dehydration and its potential impact also seems to be much underestimated, especially where people are drinking sweet, fizzy drinks, tea and coffee, but no actual, straightforward pure water. There is some evidence to show that dehydration can be a real issue for people who have a diagnosis of bipolar disorder and who tend to drink lots of Pepsi, Coke, sugary drinks and coffee, which all cause overall water loss. This has damaging knock-on effects for our health, and many people find things tend to be much calmer once they are properly hydrated. Two studies at the University of Connecticut, reported in the *British Journal of Nutrition*, showed that even mild dehydration (defined as around 1.5 per cent loss in normal water volume in the body) caused irritability, loss of concentration, fatigue, anxiety and adverse changes in mood. While many of us have now taken on board the health message that we need to drink plenty of water every day, chlorinated tap water is not the answer. Treat yourself to a water filter or, better still, find out if you have any natural springs of drinking water in your area.

We also need to consider the toxins we take in through our skin. High street brands of shampoos and shower gels all contain parabens, which are highly toxic. Parabens-free products are available from health food stores. They are more expensive, but once you have tried them you will find that even the smell of those with chemicals seems offensive. Our health deserves the best.

Some of these changes may seem small and trivial, but as we learn to nurture ourselves in little ways so we start to do this with the bigger, life-changing issues too. If the idea of change feels too daunting despite knowing you need to make some, then start with small things that don't feel too threatening. When you come to tackle the bigger changes, you might feel you need to get support. If so, re-read Step 2 on 'Reaching out'.

As we start to get rid of the unhelpful, the toxic, we automatically start thinking about healthier alternatives. Let's take a closer look now at nurturing and supportive measures we can put in place. The crux to this is wanting to take care of ourselves, wanting to be kind and loving to ourselves. We are on a journey to healthy self-regard and self-love. This is what the 'Seven steps to healing' are all about, perhaps none more so than the next one, 'Making life changes'.

Step 6

Making life changes

'The experience was a chance to reset my life.'

Jane

Work that honours your creativity; living somewhere healing and nurturing; following your heart's calling; intimacy with a significant other; honouring your sensitivity – your psyche and your soul are longing for this positive change, for more depth and meaning to your life. As you take responsibility for your healing, as you reach out for support, find the right professionals and start to do away with the toxic, so gradually you will be able to start addressing whatever issue is most pressing for you. Gradually you will be able to make the positive life changes that in time can completely transform your life. This is what Step 6 is all about. It means nurturing and nourishing ourselves on every level; it means making changes, small and big, to support our total wellbeing. This is what healing requires. Here is just part of what it looked like for Katie, whom we met when she was working through guilt.

> I was now starting to become more interested in the body–mind connection as I couldn't help but notice how much better my own health had been since my emotions were more stable. Everything was synchronizing; body, mind and spirit. Knowing how important it was to have not only precious relaxation time in order to give my poor little brain a well-earned rest, but also time alone to enable me to listen to my soul in order to keep me on track, I booked myself a week in Crete. It was also a kind of gift to myself, time to assimilate my new knowledge and to prove that my confidence had now developed enough to allow me to go on holiday alone and actually enjoy my own company.

Where do we start?

Our priorities will depend on what we are coping with. It may be that we just need to focus on looking after ourselves and getting over the worst of the crisis. Or it may be that only some aspects of how we live need transforming. Or maybe we need to take stock and make changes in all the key areas: where we live and who we live with, where we work and who we work with.

Sometimes these changes are forced on us anyway. A significant relationship may have ended or we may have lost our job, triggering the crisis or maybe even because of our crisis. Even though this feels very painful when it happens, in time we may come to realize it was what needed to happen. If you have been in crisis recently, wait until things have settled down before making any major changes. If some changes feel very challenging, make sure you get support.

Nourishing your soul

All of these changes – following our calling, putting in place work and lifestyles that are not overly stressful, honouring our sensitivity and giving our lives more depth and meaning – for me, these all come down to nourishing ourselves at the soul level. This is the deepest level of self-care, the deepest nurturing we can give ourselves.

You may want to bring some element of spiritual practice into your day or week, however loosely you define 'spiritual'. This may be particularly so if you have been struggling with issues to do with the meaning, purpose or value of life – your life. It can help you gain a whole different perspective and help you get in touch with what you want to do with your life, what would help give it some meaning.

It may simply be that right now your number one priority is to get better, to heal on different levels. This could be a hugely valuable purpose to your life at this time. Later, when you feel ready to review this, it may lead to other priorities. Many who have been through crisis quite rightly feel they have something to offer and want to be of service in some way. This certainly helps give meaning to our life.

At the most simple level, you could just light a candle for your healing every morning when you get up, setting your intention for the day to focus on that. If you like to use prayer or affirmations, this would be a good time.

Do you like to sing? Join a choir or take up chanting, from Tibetan Buddhist chanting to mantras to the lively Hindu tradition of Kirtan, devotional and spiritual music. If you like to sing *and* dance, the Dances of Universal Peace can be a practice in their own right. Deeply soulful, they bring in simple chants and mantras, drawing on all the faiths of the world, to accompany the simple dance steps. Prayer and meditation, whether Buddhist, Christian, Sufi or other, are powerful spiritual practices. Maybe you like to read uplifting literature. I find spiritual biography and autobiography particularly inspiring. I have read and re-read the story of Dipa Ma's life. Other teachers from across the traditions include Ramana Maharishi, St Teresa of Ávila and Paramahansa Yogananda.

If you have a strong connection with nature, then you already have something in place that can nurture you at soul level. If getting out in nature really nourishes and centres you, bringing you inner peace, then make that an absolute priority.

Kindness, forgiveness and gratitude

Many faiths around the world emphasize the importance of kindness and generosity. A Buddhist meditation practice of loving kindness, called *metta*, helps cultivate this quality. Recent fascinating research has shown that kindness is very good for our mental health. Not only does it create positive physiological changes associated with happiness, it also, according to the Mental Health Foundation, helps reduce feelings such as anger, aggression and hostility which have a negative impact on our mind and body. Compassion-Focused Therapy, developed by Professor Paul Gilbert, helps those affected by trauma, for instance, to cope with shame, reduce anxiety and move from self-criticism to self-compassion.

The Buddhist *metta* practice starts with cultivating compassion towards ourselves during the first stage of the meditation. This is a great practice if we're carrying childhood wounding and need to learn to love and value ourselves. The starting point has to be kindness towards ourselves, or self-compassion. Mental health research is confirming what the Dalai Lama has been telling us all along: kindness is good for us.

Another powerful path on our spiritual journey can be forgiveness: forgiving ourselves and those we feel have harmed us in some way. We can't force this before we're ready, which is why it is a practice in its own right. When I'm struggling with what in reality is a relatively minor issue, I find the work of the Forgiveness Project helps put things into perspective. Taking its inspiration from the South African Truth and Reconciliation Commission, this charity brings together victims and perpetrators, from white supremacists to terrorists. Working for conflict resolution and reconciliation, it is grassroots social activism at its very best.

There's a lovely gratitude practice you can do as you're lying in bed at night, just about to fall asleep. List all the things, tiny and not so tiny, that you have to be thankful for from the day just gone. Send your thanks out into the ether. Fall asleep knowing that even if it was a thorny day, there were some roses too. You may discover you had a day full of roses, a veritable bouquet.

Nourishing your soul and bringing some sort of spiritual or soulful practice into your life represents a considerable and powerful life change. It can only have a positive impact on your healing.

Intimacy

Research shows that having a loving partner cushions and protects us from the blows of life and any negative impact on our mental health. It can be hugely supportive – if it's right and if it's working. There can, however, also be great value in being single while we get to grips with our health and our lives. When we're going through the profound inner transformation of integrating psychospiritual crisis, that is enough to cope with. Once we're on track we're in a much better position to attract or create a far healthier, happier relationship. We are then likely to meet someone at our level of personal and spiritual development.

Ask yourself these questions of a potential partner:

- Does he or she have integrity?
- Is he or she committed to personal and spiritual development?
- How high is this person's self-esteem?
- Does he or she behave in a mature and responsible way?
- How open is he or she emotionally?
- Does he or she have a positive attitude towards life?

If you've had a series of painful or disastrous relationships or have never experienced life as a single person, consider consciously choosing to stay single for a while. You'll know when you've done the work, when you're ready to re-engage, this time on different terms. Or you may get to like being single so much that you decide not to bother!

Your heart's calling

Finding or creating work for ourselves that honours our sensitivity, our creativity and all we have to offer, while also paying the bills, is the ultimate goal for each of us. Ask yourself these questions:

- What do you absolutely love to do?
- What do you have to offer others?
- How do you want to be of service?
- What work would allow you to honour your sensitivity?

If you feel you are a Highly Sensitive Person (HSP, see page 80), you may well benefit from a job that enables you to work from home. A noisy open-plan office would probably be your idea of hell. Working from home enables you to be in control of your environment and the amount of contact you have with others. If you would like to work with a life coach but can't afford it, buddy up with a friend and coach each other. Or buy a life-coaching book and work through the programme. You might want to look for an author who values a holistic, spiritual approach, like Tara Mohr.

Mindfulness

Mindfulness is now being taught in schools, it's being taught in some of the leading companies in the world, such as Apple and Google, it's being taught in the health service, it's even being taught in the American army. I strongly recommend that anyone struggling with health issues incorporates it into his or her daily life. It is nothing less than a natural medicine for the mind, free from any of the toxic side effects that come with medication. Particularly if spiritual practice *per se* doesn't feel right for you, you can approach mindfulness in a totally secular way and benefit hugely. Look for a local class and check that it doesn't include Buddhist philosophy or teachings, if that's not what you want. Other practices which will help you become more mindful and inhabit your body more fully are things like yoga or chi gung. These are all great stress busters.

Honouring our sensitivity

Coping with our sensitivity is about far more than just managing stress. The more sensitive you are, the more you will benefit from having a quiet, gentle lifestyle. Chances are, if you have struggled with mental health issues, that you are fairly, if not extremely, sensitive by nature. This is not a bad thing. It does, however, need some careful thought as to how to cope with the bombardment of daily life. Elaine Aron's helpful book *The Highly Sensitive Person* includes strategies for what she terms Highly Sensitive People (HSPs). Mindfulness helps enormously here too, by helping us become aware of what is overwhelming or too grating for our level of sensitivity.

My story
For me, coping with my sensitivity has become a way of life. Over the years I've gradually made more and more adjustments towards living a quiet, gentle life, to the extent that my lifestyle now feels a bit like being on retreat most of the time. I do my best to avoid supermarkets and shopping malls. I find that public places like restaurants and coffee shops can be very noisy and jarring; given the choice, and the weather, I will always sit outside. I avoid being on the phone or using my laptop for about an hour before going to bed. My husband and I also choose not to have a television. As most of our friends have made the same choice, this doesn't seem so odd.

Delicious food

Diet, as we have seen, is increasingly being recognized as crucial to our mental health just as much as it is to our physical health. When our approach is holistic we can't separate mental health from physical health; we are one being, with all our physical, mental, energetic and emotional systems interacting. It stands to reason, then, if we want to heal we need to feed our bodies the very best we can. This means preferably organic food. Any food that is not organic could well have residues of harmful chemicals. We don't need those toxins. Ideally most of our meals will be home-cooked. This way we avoid processed food with all its additives and very little nutritional value. We can aim for this once we're well and truly over any period of crisis.

We may also be deficient in various essential vitamins or minerals and need to take supplements. Commonly people lack nutrients such as vitamin C, iodine, zinc, magnesium and essential fatty acids – in other words, omega 3, 6 and 9. Research by the London Institute of Psychiatry and Harvard Medical School has shown the benefits of essential fatty acids in treating and supporting mental health. Vegetarians and vegans are also often short of B12, which the brain needs for its wellbeing.

When under the kind of stress that comes with any crisis, especially if it is for a prolonged period, we can become severely depleted of essential nutrients. Our adrenals can also become exhausted, which in turn can impact on our thyroid. Natural remedies such as liquorice root can support the adrenals, and iodine, for instance in the form of sea kelp, can help the thyroid. With the physical and mental exhaustion or burn-out that can follow a period of high energy it is particularly important to eat well and supplement appropriately.

Fun exercise

If the word 'exercise' fills you with as much dread as it does me, then remember that fun things like dancing are excellent forms of exercise too. There is such a huge range of different kinds of dance available today, from all the classics like tango, salsa or jive to circle dancing, 5 Rhythms™, Nia and Zumba®. There is something to suit everyone and every temperament.

Also consider whether you want to get your exercise in some kind of group or class setting or whether you prefer to do something on your own or with a friend. The advantage of doing it with at least one other person is that it can help to maintain momentum if your motivation starts to flag.

When choosing a form of exercise you will enjoy and therefore will be more likely to keep up, remember that apart from the myriad dance forms there is the whole gamut of yoga, tai chi, chi gung and Pilates on offer. The list is endless, from rock climbing to circus skills and everything in between. If finances are tight, nothing beats good old-fashioned walking. Better still, get out in nature for a walk. Research has shown the benefits of exercise for mental health, especially for depression. Make it fun!

Doing the work

If you are following the seven steps, taking responsibility for your healing, reaching out for support, seeking those who validate your journey towards wholeness, finding the right health professional for you, focusing on success stories and doing away with the toxic, then you are laying the foundations for the amount of change you truly need to make. You are setting the scene for a happy and fulfilled future to be possible *and* sustainable. You can be proud. Congratulate yourself on the work you are putting into your healing. You are doing away with habits and ways of life that are not supportive and welcoming in those which are. You are radically changing the way you live your life. It is from this root and branch level of transformation that healing comes. Well done!

Step 7
Seeing crisis as a gift

'My mind was opened to a new level of awareness.'

Mary

Seeing crisis as a gift means seeing it as an opportunity, an opportunity for healing and growth, an opportunity to:

- tend to the call of psyche and soul;
- reframe our experience of crisis;
- find meaning in our lives;
- help heal future generations;
- cultivate a positive attitude;
- welcome and embrace our sensitivity;
- cultivate acceptance;
- learn to look after and nurture ourselves;
- create our reality.

These all add up to a wonderful chance to heal at the deepest level. If this is so, our struggles are a true blessing in disguise, a brave breakthrough rather than a defeating breakdown. We may well not be able to see this while in the midst of crisis, of bitter suffering; in time we can come to this place of grace. Time and again the people I meet and speak with express no regrets whatsoever for the horrors they have been through. They tell me they wouldn't change a thing. Here is Katie Mottram again, from her memoir *Mend the Gap*.

> I consider myself to be hugely lucky. Despite my doubting logical brain, I had the strength of character to listen to my soul, which led me to find a network of people in the UK Spiritual Crisis Network who understood the phenomena of spiritual emergence. With the stability of this conceptual framework to make sense of my experiences and allow natural evolution and integration, it was like coming home – the opposite of seeing psychosis as a destructive illness. I am now more able to be a 'silent witness' to my emotions, rather than letting them control me, and I have a

much more positive belief system. I know that I am on a life-long journey of learning, but it is now one I enjoy and appreciate.[15]

Tending to the call of psyche and soul

Our crisis is a message loud and clear from the depths of our being. Something is out of balance. It needs tending to. Something is damaged, wounded or simply not right and needs immediate attention. It will not wait any longer. If we do not address it now, if we do not give it the care and love that it is calling for, we may be setting ourselves up for worse later on. It's as if the psyche creates a critical situation to generate the change, the healing, we need. We can thank our crisis for alerting us to this and see it as a gift.

Reframing our experience of crisis

Right at the start of this book we saw how helpful it can be to see our mental health struggles from a different, more holistic perspective. Seeing them through a transpersonal or spiritual lens can help bring a deeper meaning to it all. This broader framework can also help give us a deeper understanding of the possible causes. This in turn can point us towards finding real, lasting healing solutions rather than simply managing symptoms.

Our mental health issues bring us the unique opportunity to reframe our experience in this validating way: that we are okay and what we are going through is okay. Not only is what we're going through okay but it is actually to be welcomed as a gift, as an opportunity to heal at the deepest level. The kind of validating possible when we approach mental health from a transpersonal perspective is all part of seeing our 'illness' as a blessing.

Finding meaning in our lives

Being out of touch with our life's calling can contribute to a mental health crisis. Our crisis is a call, an opportunity to reflect on what we really want to do with our lives. If you haven't done so already, now is the time to take stock. We can thank this tough challenge for encouraging us to do so.

Your life's calling

Key questions to ask yourself could be:

- What do you feel is the meaning or message of your crisis? What is it trying to tell you?
- What purpose does it serve for you? What higher purpose might it serve?
- Do you have a sense of being 'off track' in some way in your life?
- Why do you think you are alive?
- What is going to give meaning to your life?
- What do you feel most passionate about?
- How do you want to be of service? Who do you want to help?

Related to this is getting in touch with our creativity. We are all creative beings, and while our creativity can take myriad forms, connecting with this will help us feel really fulfilled. I'm using 'creativity' here in its broadest sense, from painting watercolours to plastering a beautifully smooth wall, from making pottery to cooking a nutritious, tasty meal. We need to find what makes our heart sing, what fills us with joy and satisfaction. A mental health crisis is a turning point in our lives, when we can take time to re-evaluate our priorities. Using the crisis to identify our creative calling in life turns it from a problem to a gift, an opportunity.

Healing for future generations

If family wounding has contributed to our mental health struggles, then the healing work we do is done for the whole family. Rather than the wounding getting passed on yet again to the next generation, we are dealing with it here and now, saving our children and grandchildren from having to grapple with the self-same issues. What an extraordinary gift to be able to give our children, even if we haven't had them yet! To some extent this impacts on our siblings too, helping them to grow and heal, sometimes in subtle ways, other times with more obvious outcomes. I'm thinking here of the amazing healing work that my brother has been able to do.

Cultivating a positive attitude

Cultivating a positive attitude may not come naturally or we may feel just too worn down by the whole experience. If you feel quite negative, the important thing is not to judge this in any way. We need loving kindness towards ourselves, a great deal of loving kindness. Beating ourselves up and being our own worst critic for being negative will only make it worse. You may find that mindfulness or CBT can help you to become more aware of your tendencies. Awareness is a huge part of beginning to turn things around. Often it is all we need to effect major change in our attitude: to notice we are not being kind to ourselves or to challenge our negative or catastrophic thinking. In this way, too, we can see the crisis as an opportunity, an opportunity to start to change our attitudes, to foster more helpful ones in place of any unhelpful or toxic ones.

Welcoming and embracing our sensitivity

As part of welcoming our mental health issues as a blessing in disguise, we can also welcome our sensitivity as a gift. Indeed, Malidoma Somé (see page 115) suggests it could be just that, a gift or ability to become a healer, in its broadest sense, that is awakening right now. Our reluctance or failure to acknowledge it may have even catalysed the crisis, drawing our attention to it. Others suggest that it could be psychic ability, our sixth sense, that is calling for attention and encouragement.

For you, embracing your sensitivity may simply be recognizing that you have different needs from other people, that you thrive in different conditions from many others. The first step is recognizing that we are more sensitive than most and then working with that creatively, adjusting our lives accordingly. To help you do that I highly recommend Elaine N. Aron's book *The Highly Sensitive Person: How to thrive when the world overwhelms you.*

Whatever welcoming and embracing your sensitivity means for you personally, thank your current crisis for alerting you to it and for compelling you to stop ignoring it.

Cultivating acceptance

While doing all we can to move towards healing, we need, at the same time, to cultivate acceptance and surrender. Acceptance does not mean being passive. There is such a fine balance between surrendering and accepting how things are while at the same time taking responsibility and moving proactively towards our healing. This is where the skill of mindfulness can be very useful in helping us notice when we are resisting 'what is'. The paradox is that while being proactive in our recovery we need to not be attached to the outcome. In order to get from A to B, we need to fully accept A. If our starting point is one of pain and distress, we need much tenderness and compassion towards ourselves and our suffering to be able to even begin to accept it. This is why it's important to include kindness meditation practices when we teach mindfulness.

Learning to look after and nurture ourselves

All seven steps have really been about learning to love and nourish ourselves, whether that's learning to manage our sublime sensitivity, learning to love ourselves enough to leave damaging or toxic relationships or jobs, or caring for our wellbeing sufficiently to want to eat a healthy diet and live somewhere nurturing. When we start doing things, however small, that show us we care about ourselves, we know we have turned an important corner. We are starting to see ourselves as the precious beings we are. If our crisis has led us to this, then it has indeed been a wonderful gift. Mary says: 'Over the years I have developed more and more awareness of taking care of myself, validating my feelings, understanding and compassion for myself and others.'

Creating our reality

We are what we believe. The more we believe in our ability to heal, the more we create that. We can literally create our healing, our path to wholeness. Don't let anybody tell you otherwise. Each of us has access to infinite creativity. If we direct that towards our healing there is no stopping us. This is part of the gift, the opportunity we have been given. My hope is that you are now ready to see your crisis as a gift. From there you can create your own personal healing journey, following each of the seven steps.

So many grapple with mental health issues. As more and more of us move towards wellbeing, offering our talents to the world, I believe there is nothing that will make a greater difference to the collective good, to our collective wellbeing. As more and more people wake up to the deeper calling of their psyche and soul, the world will become a different place, a better place. Anything you do in your life is not just for you but also for the greater good, to show others what is possible.

From the depths of my being, I wish you well on your journey to health, wholeness and happiness.

Part 3
HEALING APPROACHES

4

Therapy and mindfulness

Towards integrative mental health care

Now that we've embraced the 'Seven steps to healing', let's take a look at some of the healing approaches you might want to engage with on your journey to wholeness and health.

Each person's healing journey is unique. It is a personal blend of therapies and practices based on individual needs. Often, through psychiatric care, we are offered only one solution, medication. We have already started to see the treasure chest of other healing possibilities. Each can be used alongside prescribed drugs, creating the very best of integrative mental health care. In exactly the same way, many cancer patients alleviate the side effects of chemotherapy and surgery by using natural remedies and dietary supplements. They may also work to heal any emotional and psychological causes of their illness, eliminate toxicity from their diets and their lives and make any radical lifestyle changes they need to. All this alongside their regular oncology appointments. This is known as an 'integrative' approach to health care. These principles apply equally to mental health.

In the process of creating our personal package of integrative care we need to be prepared to go slightly off-piste, to try new things in our search for what works for each one of us as individuals. Several of the healing approaches we explore in this chapter and the next have been central to my own healing journey, in particular psychotherapy and mindfulness. Bear in mind that different approaches are right for different people; trust your intuition.

Talking therapies

There are myriad types of counselling and psychotherapy, but for our purposes we will focus mainly on those which consciously include the spiritual dimension. A broad distinction between counselling and psychotherapy is that usually counselling is shorter term and consequently does not go as deep as psychotherapy. For this reason they serve different purposes and suit different situations. The crucial issue of how to find a good counsellor or therapist is addressed in Step 3, 'Finding the right healthcare professional'.

Engaging in any talking therapy is a brave thing to do. Working through our wounding can be very painful, though enormously rewarding. It is also no small undertaking because of the financial commitment involved. Often trainee counsellors and therapists charge lower rates. They also usually have more supervision until they are fully qualified.

The talking therapies available free of charge on the UK National Health Service (NHS) tend, in my experience, to be limited, in both scope and duration, as well as sometimes having very long waiting lists. Something like six weeks of CBT can, however, serve as a good starting point. Your GP should be able to refer you to psychology services. If you are struggling with specific issues, such as bereavement, sexual abuse or domestic violence, you can often access counselling free of charge. This might be through your local hospice or women's shelter or through national charities such as Cruse. If you can't find what you're looking for, ask your GP.

My story
Despite all the tears, I feel I gained immeasurably from the one-to-one therapy I had with a transpersonal therapist. My sense of self was strengthened, as were my personal boundaries. I learnt not to accept abusive behaviour, behaviour I had not even recognized as such, having grown up in an abusive household. It had simply been the norm. From having had a somewhat damaged ego, I moved to a place of having a much healthier and stronger psyche. Along the way there were major healing crises, like the one I have described in Egypt in 2003. My therapist held and supported me through these, being as much spiritual mentor and director to me as therapist. That served me very well.

If you can afford to invest in your health in this way and find the right therapist for you, counselling or psychotherapy can be enormously healing and enriching. If you particularly want to explore dreams and any mythical, archetypal themes coming up for you, then a Jungian approach might suit you. It does not necessarily have to be traditional Jungian analysis. Many therapists today combine different schools of training and draw on different influences and traditions. Let's take a look at a few approaches in more detail.

Psychosynthesis

Developed by the Italian Roberto Assagioli in the early 1900s, this psychotherapy works towards the 'synthesis' of the whole person, bringing together the different parts of ourselves, including our spiritual Self. What makes this synthesis possible is that part of us which is the observer, the witness. Assagioli identified three aims of psychosynthesis: 'harmonious inner integration, true Self-realization, and right relationships with others'.

Self-realization for Assagioli meant an evolution of consciousness, leading to ever higher, more expanded levels of consciousness and ultimate union with the universal Self. A strength of psychosynthesis is that Assagioli, having worked as a psychiatrist, understood the process of spiritual emergence and emergency. In his paper 'Self-realization and psychological disturbances' he wrote about the kind of psychospiritual crisis we can go through as we move towards full realization of the Self.

Today, psychosynthesis makes a very useful therapeutic approach for anyone wanting transpersonal help with their mental health struggles because it includes this understanding of spiritual emergency.

Core Process psychotherapy

Core Process psychotherapy was developed by the Karuna Institute in Devon, founded by Maura Sills. Drawing on the best of many approaches, it brings together transpersonal psychology, developmental psychology and body psychotherapy. The principles of Buddhism, such as mindfulness (present moment awareness) and *metta* (loving kindness) underpin the whole.

Core Process therapists are trained to have an awareness of spiritual emergence and emergency. Indeed, this is where I first came across the term, when I was doing a course with Karuna as part of my healing journey. I was fortunate to find a Core Process therapist who had personal experience of going through psychospiritual crisis. This helped enormously when I found myself in crisis during the first year of training. It is not uncommon for those training, whether in psychosynthesis, Core Process or another approach, to go through a personal healing crisis because of the depth of the work.

You do not have to have Buddhist leanings to benefit from Core Process psychotherapy. Many therapists find that most of their clients are not Buddhists and sessions are not conducted with any particular reference to Buddhism. The Karuna Institute holds a directory of Core Process therapists around the UK and beyond.

Family constellations

A family approach which can bring lasting resolution is family constellations. As so much of our wounding can come from our families of origin, sometimes down through generations, family constellations can be powerfully therapeutic. Developed in Germany by Bert Hellinger, constellation work has proved popular in numerous countries around the world, with many now trained and qualified to lead sessions. Along with family systems theory, Hellinger brought in elements of psychodrama and ancestral healing. Having lived in Africa for many years, he saw how native Africans had a far stronger connection with their ancestors. Ancestors were at the centre of their lives and rituals, experienced in a positive way.

When taking part in a constellation you can have the role of participant observer where you may be called on to play a family member. Alternatively, if your own constellation is being played out, you choose which members of the group you want to represent your family, including choosing someone to be 'you', to represent yourself. You then watch as the constellation unfolds, guided by the facilitator. At a certain point you are called on to step into the constellation, to replace the person playing yourself so as to be at the heart of the constellation for its final unfolding. This wonderful process taps into the energy field of the particular family, bringing insight and heart-felt change.

My story
My personal experience with family constellations first came as an observer. Later I had the opportunity to set up and take part in a couple of constellations about my own family. I had the privilege of working with Christoph Greatorex, a highly experienced and skilful constellation leader. The most moving work I ever did with him was when he led workshops for recovering alcoholics from a rehabilitation centre. As this

was a group of men, Christoph was looking for female volunteers to take part. It helps if women can play the roles of mothers, sisters, grand-mothers, aunts and so forth. The healing I witnessed in those workshops was phenomenal.

Once, I was invited to play the mother of the man whose constella-tion it was. In the final resolution, he knelt on his knees before me to represent the child–mother relationship. As the closing piece unfolded, I held him in my arms. He sobbed as he experienced being held by his 'mother'. Seeing big, strapping men willing to be vulnerable enough to allow the tears to flow in the service of healing is extraordinary. It was also very healing for me, having had an alcoholic father, to see that it is possible to recover from such addictions and the underlying wounding. Anything is possible where there is a willingness and the right support.

Open Dialogue

This therapeutic approach was developed in Finland in the 1980s to combat the country's high levels of schizophrenia. There, psych-iatric services in west Lapland have created a remarkable success story, using a form of family therapy known as Open Dialogue. This approach focuses on supporting the individual at home, within his or her network of family and friends, and encouraging all parties to work through mental health crisis with a minimum of medication.

The wider family is involved in sessions where the emphasis is on allowing each person to be heard in a non-hierarchical way. Staff, patients and family members come together as equals to explore solutions. The focus is on supporting the individual and normal-izing the experience of crisis.

Research shows that over 80 per cent of those treated with Open Dialogue return to work or their studies, and over 75 per cent show no remaining signs of 'psychosis'. These and other good outcomes are described in a study by Dr Jaako Seikkula and colleagues from the University of Jyvaskyla.[16]

Open Dialogue, thanks to the excellent results achieved, is now being introduced in many countries including the UK. It has even inspired a critically acclaimed stage play, *The Eradication of Schizophrenia in Western Lapland*, by British theatre company Ridiculusmus.

Meditation and mindfulness

In 1967, R.D. Laing travelled to Sri Lanka to study meditation and Buddhism, meditating all day every day for five months. He wasn't unique. Many travelled to India, Burma, Thailand and other countries during the 1960s for the same reason. Even the Beatles, role models to a whole generation, courted the Maharishi, founder of Transcendental Meditation (TM).

At the same time, prominent Eastern teachers made their way to the West. It was a time of great opening when teachings which had previously been available only to the few became accessible to the many. The Chinese invasion of Tibet ironically contributed to this as many Buddhist Tibetans fled the country, bringing their wisdom and understanding with them.

Of the many Eastern practices which have since become integrated into our culture, it is appropriate for us to focus on meditation and mindfulness, as they are increasingly being used in mainstream mental health care. Most people have heard of meditation, but unless we have actually experienced it, it is difficult to grasp just how soothing it can be to mind, body and soul. For those new to meditation, often the first thing they notice, as they sit quiet and still on a chair or cushion, is just how very chatty the mind is. It can come as something of a shock to hear all the endless natter, all the planning and the plotting, the criticizing and the craving. On and on and on. Gradually we learn to watch the mind in all its carryings-on and, little by little, as we observe its meanderings, it starts to settle. From these first steps in self-awareness comes all manner of self-knowledge and self-understanding.

I like to think of mindfulness as meditation's twin; they are inseparable. Both involve awareness, awareness of our thoughts, emotions and physical sensations. Their relationship is such that the awareness we learn and cultivate while sitting on the meditation cushion we then take with us through the day, into doing all our daily activities with mindful awareness. Our whole day, indeed our whole life, can then become one of practising awareness, practising mindfulness. Dipa Ma, a Buddhist teacher, said simply, 'Whatever you are doing, be aware of it.'

My story

After my spell in hospital, I faced my next major challenge 12 years later when my first husband and I split up. At the time I was lecturing full-time and doing a PhD part-time, and I had a very difficult working relationship with my head of department. With the breakdown of my marriage on top of all that, the stress was really piling up and I needed to take action. I certainly didn't want to end up in hospital again. At that point I decided, under the guidance of a psychiatrist, to take medication as a preventative measure.

I lasted two days. I couldn't think straight. It was like trying to see through the most dense fog imaginable – but trying to think through it rather than see through it. There was absolutely no way I could teach, write lectures or mark essays with that in my system. This, however, left me vulnerable to the stress that was becoming unmanageable. The situation wasn't sustainable.

That's when I discovered this natural medicine for the mind: meditation. I saw an advert for classes and, having heard that meditation was supposed to be good for stress, signed up. This was a small, simple decision but it changed my life for ever. I soon discovered there was much more to meditation than simply a powerful tool to help cope with stress.

Thanks to the pioneering work of Jon Kabat-Zinn in the United States, meditation and mindfulness have now well and truly entered mainstream medicine and are becoming integrated into it. On the mental health side, depression, eating disorders and the wounding known as 'personality disorders' are just some of the issues being alleviated by mindfulness practice.

Mindfulness-based Stress Reduction (MBSR) was developed by Kabat-Zinn. Other relevant therapies are cognitive behavioural therapy (CBT) and dialectical behaviour therapy (DBT). CBT includes the principle of mindfulness, of self-awareness, and works by helping clients become aware of the relationship between particular thoughts and feelings. For example, catastrophizing thoughts, picturing the worst possible outcome or scenario, tend to increase fear and anxiety levels. With mindful awareness we can identify when the mind is starting to catastrophize and thereby help interrupt the impact it could have emotionally. In dialectical behaviour therapy (DBT), mindfulness is even more of a central concept. Clients are specifically taught mindfulness techniques during group sessions.

Mindfulness brings with it increased self-awareness and self-knowledge, and with that comes increased self-compassion. It changes our relationship to our suffering, helping us to start loosening its grip. One distinct advantage of the practice is that for those not interested in a spiritual approach to their healing, it can be taught in a totally secular way. Indeed, this is how it is being used within the health sector, with therapies such as CBT, DBT and MBSR. This use of mindfulness is a major positive development within orthodox mental health care.

On a personal level, mindfulness has helped me through two periods of acute psychospiritual crisis: in 2003, when I ended up in a wheelchair for a few days, and again in 2006. I was so impressed with how beneficial it is in such acute situations, as opposed just to chronic ones, that in 2007 I trained to become an accredited mindfulness trainer. For me this is a way of integrating it fully into my daily life, to ensure I continue to reap the benefits. It also means I am able to offer to others a method which never fails to get results. This is true even, for example, with soldiers returning from Iraq and Afghanistan suffering from a debilitating combination of mental health issues and physical pain. As I witness that over and over again, I am in awe of mindfulness. It is an approach I profoundly believe in.

Having trained some NHS dialectical behaviour therapists in mindfulness, I saw a particular issue which in time could undermine the positive results. To be effective in our therapeutic use of mindfulness, we need to have our own daily mindfulness practice. Where staff do not take that on board, the results are likely to be watered down. It would be a great shame if this came to reflect negatively on mindfulness itself.

It is such a simple yet powerful approach, one which lends itself perfectly to self-help and to the self-management of any mental health condition. I highly recommend learning mindfulness and integrating it into your life. Be aware, however, that you need to learn at a time when you are not in crisis. As well as being a potent self-awareness tool to help you manage your mental health, it can also be a spiritual practice. As such it is best to learn mindfulness when things are relatively settled, as any spiritual practice can have the effect of heightening psychospiritual crisis.

In this chapter we have looked at several talking therapies and we have seen how a gentle yet powerful practice such as meditation can be a natural medicine for the mind. We have also seen how it is being incorporated into mainstream mental health care through the use of mindfulness.

Mindfulness is not the only practice to come to us from the East. Eastern spiritual systems and practices were, and continue to be, a significant influence on the whole transpersonal field and are at the root of many holistic therapies widely practised today. Increasingly, some of these, such as acupuncture and shiatsu, are also being integrated into orthodox treatment. Let's turn our attention now to these forms of energy medicine, as well as homeopathy, nutrition and medication.

5

More healing approaches

We have seen how teachings from the East bring us gentle yet powerful healing modalities. Meditation, which comes from Eastern Buddhism, is a wonderful natural medicine for the mind, and a potent tool for self-awareness and self-compassion. These are crucial for any healing to take place. Many people find other Eastern techniques helpful, such as acupuncture and shiatsu, which are thought to work with the body's energy channels or meridians, balancing and healing at the energetic level. All these approaches go beyond the nuts and bolts of biology and chemistry, working with subtle aspects of our bodies and our psyches.

Energy medicine

Another important influence from the East is our whole understanding of energy medicine or energy healing. Energy medicine views the physical body as surrounded by an electromagnetic field. This can be polluted or damaged by many things. On the mild end of the spectrum, it's thought that our energy field can be adversely impacted by electromagnetic pollution such as mobile telephone masts or wireless computer use. On the severe end, our energy field may be viewed as damaged by physical or emotional trauma and abuse, or by substance misuse. A combination of these, such as some sort of childhood abuse or trauma coupled with later use of cannabis, for instance, can be a perilous precursor to serious psychospiritual crisis. Whether you take the concept of the energy field literally or view it as a metaphor for our natural sensitivity, it can be seen as a useful gauge; a gauge for looking after ourselves, for knowing our limits, for protecting and respecting our boundaries, boundaries which can become extremely porous in times of crisis.

As well as the energy field around the body, energy medicine also considers that we have energy or 'chi' moving through the body, along energy channels known as meridians. Healing approaches such as acupuncture and shiatsu are said to work with these meridians to rebalance energies and help move blocked or stagnant energy. Acupuncture, in particular auricular acupuncture (of the ear), is recognized as helping with addiction issues. It is recommended by the UK Department of Health for detox purposes and is well documented in the medical literature for a variety of healing purposes.

Shiatsu is similar to acupuncture, but instead of needles, gentle pressure is applied by hand on energy or *tsubo* points. To describe it as a cross between acupuncture and massage probably doesn't do justice to this wonderfully soothing and rebalancing therapy. Today, shiatsu is being offered on psychiatric wards, such as the highly respected Maudsley Hospital in London.

Char Scrivener worked as a shiatsu therapist for one of the UK Mental Health Trusts at a project for people with 'long-term mental health problems'. The people she worked with had diagnostic labels ranging from schizophrenia and bipolar to personality disorder. Those referred by the Refugee Support Service within the Trust also suffered additionally from post-traumatic stress, having been 'tortured, raped, witnessed close members of their families killed in front of them' and more. In a paper presented to a European Shiatsu Congress, available from the UK Shiatsu Society, she tells the following story of one young woman's remarkable journey of healing.

> . . . a few months after I had started working at the project, 'L', a young woman, was referred for Shiatsu. She had a medical diagnosis of Multiple Disassociative Personality Disorder (MDPD), had been periodically hospitalised and had been on all sorts of medication . . .
>
> When she started having Shiatsu with me she had come off medication . . . She was under the care of a psychiatrist but also seeing a psychotherapist working at the hospital . . . One day in the Shiatsu session L went into a personality she referred to as animal, she started snarling, clawing the ground and moving around like a caged animal . . .
>
> I didn't know what to do, the one thing I managed to do was keep my hand on her and say 'it's OK, I'm here, you can come back if you want' something like that, I just didn't know what else to do . . . one minute I was rotating her shoulder and the next she was the wild beast.

Gradually she came back; I can't remember what happened in the rest of the session, we basically picked ourselves up, brushed ourselves down and started all over again as 'normal' people.

. . . Ultimately what was important was that I managed to keep contact both physically and verbally, I did hold a space – for both of us. A day or two later L's psychotherapist phoned me. Both L and he felt that this had been a very important and positive thing for L as she usually only went into this personality when she felt extremely threatened, and she didn't feel threatened with me, on the contrary she felt very safe with me. Therefore this was a good sign, there was a change. There was a space where she felt safe to go into that persona which would normally only manifest in a completely opposite situation . . .

Over a period of about seven years, L re-integrated, she still had a psychiatric diagnosis but it was no longer DMPD. She has taken various courses, is doing work experience and getting out into the local community more. Seven years may seem a long time but in relation to the process she undertook to disassociate it was relatively short and it was very much a process she engaged with and actually led.[17]

As L's is a story of such severe wounding, it illustrates very powerfully what energy healing such as shiatsu can achieve with the right combination of psychotherapy and psychiatric support alongside. As we discussed in Step 3, it is, however, essential to work with an accredited and trustworthy practitioner (see page 57).

Somebody else who has a great deal of experience of working with shiatsu in a mental health setting is Katharine Hall. She worked on acute admissions and recovery wards for two UK Health Trusts, most notably at the Maudsley Hospital in London. Her clients covered the full spectrum of psychiatric labels, ranging from depression and anxiety through to psychosis and schizophrenia, including issues such as feeling suicidal and self-harming. They reported the following benefits from shiatsu:

- feeling more relaxed
- fresh hope and new perspective
- better confidence
- increased sense of power in their situation
- appreciation of the individual time
- appreciation of the quiet time off the ward

- liking the opportunity of treatment continuity (many return to hospital shiatsu sessions as outpatients).[18]

Both shiatsu and acupuncture are based on the premise that there is no separation between body and mind. In Traditional Chinese Medicine (TCM), which they stem from, there is no concept of mental 'illness' existing without physical imbalance. Therapists aim to access the mental through the chi, or life force energy, of the physical body. Acupuncture is commonly used to treat psychiatric issues in China, usually every other day for three to six months. For mania, twice daily treatments are used for a shorter period. This is because 'Heart Fire Effulgence' episodes, which is how mania is seen in TCM terms, are generally found to last 12 hours, but at any rate rarely longer than a week.[19]

As you can see, there are different ways to approach energy healing. A truly holistic approach to our mental health must encompass an understanding of, and sensitivity to, this vital energetic level of our beings.

Other healing methods

Herbalism and homeopathy, ayurveda and anthroposophy: these are some of the healing approaches which are complete systems of medicine in their own right, in the same way as Traditional Chinese Medicine. They are holistic and address all levels of our being. While it is beyond our scope here to look in detail at all these, increasingly research shows the benefits of such systems of medicine for mental health. Practitioners may be interested, for example, in research-based texts such as Lake and Spiegel's *Complementary and Alternative Treatments in Mental Health Care*. For our purposes I would like to focus particularly on homeopathy and nutritional medicine.

Homeopathy

Homeopathy is the second largest system of medicine in the world, according to the World Health Organization, with a large research evidence base showing its effectiveness. This includes meta-analysis studies, where the results of clinical trials are pooled and overall findings analysed (see the Homeopathy Research Institute website).

A landmark Swiss report by Bornhoft and Matthiessen, translated into English as *Homeopathy in Healthcare: Effectiveness, appropriateness, safety, costs*, thoroughly reviews the scientific literature and ends:

> In conclusion we have established that there is sufficient supporting evidence for the pre-clinical (experimental) as well as clinical effects of homeopathy, and that in absolute terms, as well as when compared to conventional therapies, it offers a safe and cost-effective treatment.

While there has long been evidence that homeopathy can be beneficial for both physical and psychological conditions, what has perhaps been lacking until more recently is a scientific explanation of how it works. Homeopath Peter Adams, who has been practising for 30 years, has taken an interest in this. His most recent book is *Homeopathy: Good science – how new science validates homeopathy*. He outlines how the new science of complex systems is now showing homeopathy's holistic view of the human organism to be valid. New science is also explaining how the remedies work. Homeopathic remedies are made from dilutions of medicinal substances in water. The greater the dilution, the more potent the remedy. Leading edge science is now proving, Adams tells us, that water can hold information, that it can hold a 'memory'. This is thanks to its highly unusual molecular structure that can retain an imprint of what has been dissolved in it.

Masaru Emoto's research into the properties of water caught the public's imagination with his superb photographs of crystals formed in frozen water. In his book *Hidden Messages in Water*, a *New York Times* best seller, Emoto reports finding that water exposed to loving thoughts and vibrations shows bright, complex and colourful crystalline patterns, while water exposed to negative thoughts and vibrations forms incomplete, asymmetrical patterns with dull colours. His research, published in the *Journal of Alternative and Complementary Medicine*, and his books have brought to public awareness the fact that water can be programmed with specific vibrations. In much the same way, in homeopathy the imprint of a medicinal substance remains in water even after the substance itself has been so diluted as to no longer be physically present.

Homeopathy treats the whole person and the individual person. Finding the right remedy is very much based on the individual and the symptoms specific to that person. As a result two people presenting with, for example, depression will not necessarily benefit from the same remedy. This is shown by the following two case studies.

A man aged 54 has recurrent depression in a cycle of two or three days every few weeks. He becomes debilitated and unable to cope – with the feeling of falling off a cliff. He gets aching limbs and weakness, where it is an effort to move, and he feels despairing. He normally thrives on deadlines and stress but when depressed is needy and submissive. He took the remedy *pulsatilla* 10m. With the next bout of depression he felt a little more control than usual. Two months later he said the treatment had been successful. That was eleven years ago and the depression has never been as severe since.[20]

A woman suffers from periodic depressions. She experiences many of the common symptoms of depression and anxiety, but also she can feel guilty and very angry against herself for no longer being able to cope, and intolerant of others. She cannot abide pity and prefers to be hard-working. Often her problems are much worse before periods. The main homeopathic remedy for self-criticism, guilt and associated depression is *aurum* . . . After each treatment with this remedy she is better, usually for several years at a time.[21]

These case studies are taken from *Homeopathy: Good science* by homeopath Peter Adams. More research into the role of homeopathy in the treatment of depression is currently being undertaken at the University of Sheffield.

In terms of the safety of homeopathy cited by the Swiss report, one distinct advantage, from the point of view of mental health, is that it can be prescribed alongside psychiatric medication.

Jonathan had long found homeopathy helpful in coping with depression which sometimes tipped over into suicidal feelings. When he had a much needed spell in his local psychiatric hospital, he wanted to be able to use homeopathy. He knew it had helped him previously and he also knew it wouldn't conflict at all with the psychiatric medication he was on. Sadly, he felt obliged to take the remedies in secret. Jonathan's concern was that staff would not allow him to take them. At the same time he felt staff didn't have the right or the authority to stop him. More recently, Jonathan has been able to use homeopathy to rebalance himself and ward off the need to spend time on the wards.

Unfortunately, homeopathy has become something of a political issue and has come under media attack in recent years. It is worth noting that one of the most outspoken opponents of this system of medicine, the organization Sense About Science, receives funding from pharmaceutical companies, who may see homeopathy as a threat to their profit margins.

While homeopathy continues to be controversial in the UK despite being available on the National Health Service (NHS), some 30,000 doctors in Germany and France prescribe it. An estimated 30 million Europeans use homeopathy. Significantly, as mentioned before, it can be used alongside psychiatric medication, for those interested in integrative mental health care.

Nutritional medicine

In restoring and maintaining mental health, the role of what we eat is becoming more recognized and accepted. A measure of the extent to which this has been accepted within mainstream medicine is, for example, the MSc in Nutritional Medicine, an evidence-based course for doctors, pharmacists and other health professionals, offered by the University of Surrey.

Nutritional medicine, also known as orthomolecular medicine, is, however, biochemical in nature. While much of the nutritional guidance is valid and valuable, it tells only part of the story. Many orthomolecular practitioners take as their starting point the idea that mental health struggles are caused by a biochemical imbalance. The transpersonal approach is more holistic. It considers mind, body *and* spirit, rather than simply biochemistry. A holistic nutritional approach which does encompass the spiritual dimension is, rather confusingly, called biological medicine. In other words, there are two distinct approaches to nutrition, the orthomolecular, which is biochemical, and the biological, which is more holistic.

Malnutrition

Our eating and drinking habits may threaten our mental wellbeing. Some research has shown that soft drinks are linked with depression. A ten-year study investigated the drinking habits of 265,000 people and found that those who drank more than four cans of soft drinks a day were 30 per cent more likely to experience depression than those who drank none, with the risk being apparently greater with diet drinks. The findings were presented to the American Academy of Neurology by lead researcher Dr Honglei Chen of the National Institutes of Health in North Carolina.

As a population, owing to the processed, non-organic foods we eat, we tend to be deficient in many essential minerals, vitamins and nutrients. The most common ones are zinc, magnesium, iodine and essential fatty acids. Interestingly, magnesium was commonly used as a mood stabilizer before the Second World War.

We can call this 'affluent malnutrition'; we may be relatively wealthy yet our diets are impoverished. Such poor diets are rampant in our Western society, so rampant that in the United States they are referred to as SAD (Standard American Diet). This malnutrition is particularly widespread among mental health sufferers. SAD typically consists of a high intake of red meat, processed foods, refined grains and sugary and high-fat foods. It's perhaps no coincidence that Standard American Diet's initials are the same as those of Seasonal Affective Disorder, a debilitating form of depression that typically strikes in winter when light levels are low.

Gut dysbiosis, a bacterial imbalance in the gut, and accompanying toxicity are also remarkably common yet go largely undetected and undiagnosed, as conventional medicine tends not to recognize yeast overgrowth as a health problem. Caused by such things as widespread use of antibiotics and diets high in sugar, which feeds the yeast, gut dysbiosis has been linked with both physical and mental health issues because of the potent toxins it releases into the gut and the body. These issues include chronic fatigue, IBS and digestive problems, skin problems, and lowered resistance to infection on the physical side (for more on this, see *Coping with Candida* by Shirley Trickett, Sheldon Press, 2012). On the mental health side, the work of Dr William Crook, Dr Natasha Campbell-McBride, neurologist, neurosurgeon and nutritionist, and others has linked gut dysbiosis with depression, schizophrenia and autism. As we have seen, from the holistic perspective it is not possible to separate out the physical from the mental.

It can be difficult to change our entrenched habits of eating. You may find it easier if you aim to make small changes over several weeks. Many people find that by making overall changes to their diet, their mental health improves significantly over a period of months and they are able to reduce any medication – though this should be undertaken with your doctor rather than on your own.

Abram Hoffer, a Canadian biochemist and psychiatrist, claimed success rates as high as 80 per cent treating schizophrenics with a nutritional approach for over 50 years. He measured recovery by 'freedom from symptoms, ability to socialize with family and friends and paying income tax'. Hoffer expected his patients to do well because that was what he saw time and again, and he gave them that confidence. So it seems likely that his positive results were to do with more than simply nutrition; he was giving his patients positive, validating messages. He also used psychiatric drugs sparingly.

Medication

Few things are more contentious or emotive within the mental health field than medication. My recent experience at a social event neatly sums up the dichotomy.

I attended a lunch with writing colleagues, where invariably the conversation turns to whatever book we're currently working on. One woman, when I mentioned mental health, talked about anti-depressants causing suicidal thoughts as a side effect. She was obviously familiar with the scandal surrounding Prozac. In Germany, Prozac was initially rejected by the German drug licensing authority, Bundesgesundheitsamt (BGA), as 'completely unsuitable for the treatment of depression'. In the United States, there have been court cases against the manufacturer, Eli Lilly.

Then, within minutes, I spoke to another person, a successful non-fiction author who makes a good living from her writing. When I mentioned mental health this time, the woman told me she is bipolar and has been taking lithium for years. She was clear that her career success and her ability to get on with her life were thanks to that.

How many of us, when faced with the tough decision of whether to take medication or not, have access to all the information we need to make an informed, balanced choice? How many of us, whether it is for ourselves or for a loved one, actually know the full facts around the risk–benefit ratio of psychiatric drugs? Precious few, I suspect. Thanks to the work of Robert Whitaker and others, more and more of us are becoming better informed.

Chemical imbalance: a myth?

In his award-winning book *Anatomy of an Epidemic*, Whitaker, an investigative journalist, charts the history of psychiatry. He explores decades of mainstream research, showing how drugs commonly used today as anti-depressants and anti-psychotics were originally discovered by chance, developed from such unlikely sources as chemical dyes and muscle relaxants. These compounds seemed to alleviate some symptoms, so researchers then set about trying to explain how they worked. This is where the theory of chemical imbalance in the brain came from. Whitaker shows how the work of Schildkraut and van Rossum, who originally postulated the theory, was based on flawed research.

These ideas are not new but have been largely ignored or dismissed up to now. As early as the year 2000 Joseph Glenmullen, clinical instructor in psychiatry at Harvard Medical School, wrote in *Prozac Backlash*:

> Through the 1970s and 1980s a curious circularity invaded psychiatry, as 'diseases' began to be 'modeled' on the medications that 'treat' them. If a drug elevated serotonin in test tubes, then it was presumptuously argued that patients helped by the medication must have serotonin deficiencies even though we lack scientific proof for the idea.[22]

Stanford psychiatrist David Burns, quoted by Whitaker, also dismisses the low-serotonin theory of depression: 'I spent the first several years of my career doing full-time research on brain serotonin metabolism, but I never saw any convincing evidence that any psychiatric disorder, including depression, results from a deficiency of brain serotonin.'

The scenario portrayed by such psychiatrists, through their extensive research, is that there is no proof that mental health issues are caused by chemical imbalances in the brain. So is the chemical imbalance theory of mental 'illness' a myth? This is difficult to believe or accept. The chemical imbalance theory has been so drummed into us that everybody knows it to be true. It's a fact. Isn't it? But Whitaker, drawing on peer-reviewed research papers, thoroughly and precisely shows not only how this myth was created but also how it has been maintained. Psychiatric theories of chemical imbalance start to look more like a medical anachronism than medical accuracy.

There are many powerful interests in perpetuating the myth, not least the pharmaceutical companies. As Whitaker shows, anything which threatens drug revenues tends to be dismissed as quackery. Yet most research into psychiatric drugs is carried out by the very same pharmaceutical companies who then manufacture and sell those drugs. There are instances where it has been proven in a court of law that the researchers (i.e. the pharmaceutical companies) have overstated the benefits and underplayed the risks.

Medication is not risk free. This is what Whitaker highlights. Yes, in a crisis situation it can be life-saving, but if used long term it can become life-threatening. The research he lines up showing the long-term damage caused by medication is disturbing and the life expectancy of those taking psychiatric drugs is considerably shorter than average.

So if medication can be beneficial in the short term to help us through a crisis, but dangerous when used longer term, where does that leave us? Not taking medication? Doesn't that go against everything we know and are told? Wouldn't *that* be madness? On the contrary, there are studies suggesting the benefits of keeping medication to a minimum or even not using it at all. These studies show a very different picture from conventional psychiatry. They tell of better recovery rates, fewer people ending up on disability income, more people able to live full and rich lives.

Using medication sparingly

Cross-cultural studies on schizophrenia by the World Health Organization have been widely reported. What WHO found was that outcomes were considerably better in the developing countries it studied than in the United States or some European countries. As Whitaker reports:

At the end of two years, nearly two-thirds of the patients in the 'developing countries' had had good outcomes, and slightly more than one-third had become chronically ill. In the rich countries, only 37 percent of the patients had good outcomes, and 59 percent became chronically ill.[23]

This could be attributed to many factors, but what is particularly interesting is that only '16 percent of the patients in the poor countries were regularly maintained on antipsychotics, versus 61 percent of the patients in the rich countries'. What is more, 'in Agra, India, where patients arguably fared the best, only 3 percent of the patients were kept on an antipsychotic'.

This is consistent with outcomes reported by Loren Mosher, head of schizophrenia studies at the American National Institute of Mental Health (NIMH). Mosher believed that with the right support and empathy it is possible to successfully move through an initial 'psychosis'. He established Soteria, a safe house, in California during the 1970s. His research found that at the end of two years, Soteria patients had 'lower psychopathology scores, fewer [hospital] readmissions, and better global adjustment' than a matched cohort of hospitalized patients treated with drugs. Of Soteria patients, 42 per cent had never been exposed to drugs, 39 per cent had taken them temporarily and 19 per cent had used them during the whole two-year follow-up.

In fact, Soteria safe houses had a well-documented success rate showing that 85–90 per cent of 'acute sufferers' were able to return to the community and did not suffer relapse.[24]

John Weir Perry was another American psychiatrist doing similar research during the 1970s. He founded Diabasis (see page 24) and his findings tell much the same story as Mosher's, again with minimum use of psychiatric drugs. The emphasis was on supporting the individual to move through a psychotic crisis to a higher level of functioning – in other words, to heal and grow. Perry reported the results of outcome studies and a three-year follow-up in his book *Trials of the Visionary Mind*. The results showed patients treated without medication did much better, in terms of recurrence of 'psychosis' and emotional development, than those treated with drugs.

As mentioned earlier in this chapter, Abram Hoffer, who treated schizophrenics for 50 years with nutritional medicine, claimed his good recovery rates were thanks to nutritional supplements, and he also used medication sparingly. The very fact that he expected his patients to do well and communicated that to them will have contributed to recovery rates.

This kind of spoken validation has also been found to be an important factor by mental health services in Finland, where Open Dialogue was developed. Seeing patients do well with this particular approach, staff are able to reassure them, telling them they will be okay. In the staff's experience, giving people this positive message of hope makes a huge difference to outcomes.

Staff here do not prescribe drugs in the first instance. They have learnt that for those presenting with their first episode, this gives the opportunity for spontaneous recovery, without interference. They find that people are far more likely to be able to get on with their lives, studying, working and so forth, than if they are medicated.

What all this research has in common is that each study shows a positive correlation between keeping drug use to a minimum and good outcomes. Keeping drugs to a minimum, though, is by no means enough on its own. Validating a person's experience, giving him or her a sense that this is okay, 'you can and will come through it fine, just as many others have before you', is also crucially important. Equally vital is a therapeutic programme which supports deep healing. This is what the American psychiatrists mentioned and the Open Dialogue teams have provided. In human terms, these good outcomes mean less suffering and more people able to live the lives they hoped for. We have already looked at these crucial issues of validation and support in Step 2 of our 'Seven steps to healing' (see page 44).

A balanced approach

So often medication is the default, taken for granted as the standard treatment. I want you to know that it doesn't have to be. I'm not saying psychiatric drugs are bad or wrong; I'm saying it's a complex issue and I'm saying you need to be well informed to be able to make your own decisions.

In Part 2 you read personal success stories: people like Ursula, who takes a maintenance level of medication, and Hamilton, who is tapering off a cocktail of drugs very gradually with full medical support and supervision. You have options. That is what these stories show you. When it comes to medication, there is no one right way, no one wrong way. We each have to work out what is best for us. Each person's circumstances are unique.

While Whitaker's work is hard hitting and causing shock waves within the mental health field, its main value, I feel, is in offering a counter-balance to all those psychiatrists who from their position of authority prescribe drugs to vulnerable patients without fully discussing risks and side effects. It also seems to be encouraging some psychiatrists themselves to question over-reliance on medication and to look for alternatives such as Open Dialogue therapy.

However, do not withdraw from medication suddenly or without consulting your doctor. It is wise to start nutritional and other support, such as therapy, to create integrative care. Sudden unsupervised drug withdrawal can be dangerous, as it can result in withdrawal symptoms and toxicity problems.

We've been looking at some of the wide array of healing approaches you can use on their own or alongside others. In doing so you can create your personal healing journey, the very best in integrative mental health care. In the next chapter we'll explore some transpersonal approaches from different world traditions which shed further light on the causes, and therefore also on the solutions, to our mental health struggles.

6

Working with soul

In this final chapter, we're going to draw on wisdom from ancient indigenous cultures: wisdom which, to some extent, has been lost to us in the West and is now being rediscovered, reclaimed. We're going to look at what this ancient wisdom can teach us about mental health today. What does it tell us about the causes of our struggles? How does it fit into our transpersonal view of a mental health crisis as an opportunity for healing and growth, for personal transformation?

Other cultures often adopt different ways of exploring the roots of mental distress. These are approaches that challenge our Western way of thinking, approaches we can learn from and possibly even begin to absorb into the integrative style of health care we've been exploring. As Stephanie Marohn says of this wealth of traditional wisdom in *The Natural Medicine Guide to Bipolar Disorder*:

> [it] offers a view of mental disorders that is sorely lacking in the Western world and that holds the key to a whole other way of healing. Disregard of this view has led to treatment based on suppression of symptoms, rather than therapeutic methods that bring the body, mind and spirit back together.[25]

We have much to learn from traditional indigenous healing practices. While we can only offer a brief introduction here, many offer a transpersonal therapeutic understanding beyond the clinical. This can help us make more sense of our experience and explore deeper healing.

Psychosis or spiritual awakening?

What our society deems 'mental illness' indigenous peoples can see as an altered state of consciousness and indicative of spiritual awakening. It was filming indigenous tribes that first alerted anthropologist film maker Phil Borges to this striking contrast between how we in the West and how some indigenous cultures respond to the same set of behaviours in an individual. A major award-wining American photographer and writer, Phil Borges has been documenting indigenous and tribal cultures for more than 25 years. In his film *CrazyWise*, Borges looks at why a break from reality is usually labelled a 'first-episode psychosis' in Western culture, while many cultures see it as a spiritual awakening, supporting and celebrating it. The film also aims to explore questions such as:

- In our culture, what are the most effective treatments or supportive communities that an individual can turn to for help?
- Do some individuals have special healing or predictive abilities? If so . . .
- How could they use their gifts to contribute to society?

You can find details of *CrazyWise* on the website <www.crazywise film.com>.

Two contemporary authors who have written about this indigenous understanding specifically in relation to psychiatry and mental health are Olga Kharitidi and Malidoma Somé.

Olga Kharitidi

I highly recommend Kharitidi's book *Entering the Circle*. Kharitidi worked as a psychiatrist in a Soviet hospital and *Entering the Circle* tells of the stark life on the wards there. Set against this background, Kharitidi travels to the Siberian mountains, accompanying a friend in search of healing. As well as her outer journey to Siberia, the book charts her profound inner journey from mainstream Soviet psychiatrist to transpersonal healer. Her other books continue to explore the theme of healing trauma. Now Olga Yahontova, she works as a psychiatrist in Santa Barbara, California.

Malidoma Somé

Malidoma Somé was abducted from his native tribe, the Dagara, at the age of 4 by the Jesuits and educated in a Catholic boarding school. His book *Of Water and the Spirit* recounts how, when he returned to his tribe as an adult, he found himself a stranger, unable to speak the language and viewed with suspicion and hostility. However, the village elders decreed that he should continue to pursue a Western education and that his destiny was to impart traditional African healing wisdom to the West. Somé was then edu-cated at the Sorbonne and at Brandeis University in Massachusetts, and went on to teach at the University of Michigan.

Somé identifies several causes of mental distress from the African holistic viewpoint. One cause, he explains, is when people are not in touch with their life purpose or have strayed from it. A lack or loss of direction can result in a depressing sense of life being point-less. We see this reflected on our psychiatric wards, where many have major questions about the meaning, or purpose, of life. In a mental health crisis, this purpose is often to grow in some way to become a more evolved being or to become a healer, says Somé. He essentially views psychospiritual crisis as a wake-up call – what the Dagara call 'good news from the other world' and see as 'the birth of a healer'. If, however, this process is misunderstood and not sup-ported, it can result in behavioural and mental health issues of all kinds. It also means a vast and very sad loss of potential both for the person and for the wider community.

Becoming a healer or therapist

We can relate to the principle of this in our Western context if we think of individuals who, following a major period of psycho-spiritual crisis, feel called to train as 'healers' of some sort. This is true for so many in the health sector. I personally know massage therapists, psychologists, occupational therapists, counsellors and psychotherapists for all of whom this is the case. Having been hospitalized or experienced psychotic-type symptoms or severe depression, they have moved from breakdown to breakthrough to find their vocation in the helping professions. There are many dif-ferent kinds of healers; all are of benefit to the wider community, to us.

Healing

In Chapter 5 we touched on energy medicine and how a truly holistic approach to our mental health needs to encompass this vital energetic level of our beings. Many ancient indigenous cul-tures throughout the world use such forms of energy healing. Hands-on healing has been used for thousands of years. In Greek mythology, the great teacher Chiron's name was derived from the Greek word for hand (*kheir*), which also meant 'skilled with the hands'. Chiron taught hands-on healing to Asclepius, the god of medicine. Typically, the practitioner sees health issues as being connected to the energy body and will work to balance or return lost energy, remove negativity and return the person to renewed wholeness. Such healing works with those unseen, energetic aspects of life which affect us, including the spiritual, emotional, mental, mythical, archetypal and dream worlds.

Integrative psychiatric care

Some hospitals in Brazil provide an integrative approach where current psychiatric practices, such as medication, psychotherapy, art, music and other therapies, are employed alongside this kind of energy healing. As British psychiatrist Dr Peter Fenwick says of one of these, André Luiz Hospital in São Paulo, 'it is one of the best run mental institutions I have ever come across . . . many of the principles involved could with advantage be incorporated into psychiatric practice of other countries'.

In the foreword to Emma Bragdon's edited collection on Brazilian mental health care, psychiatrist James Lake, an authority on integrative care, writes:

> [M]ental health care is being shaped by an emerging synthesis of theories and clinical perspectives from cutting edge research in physics and the basic neurosciences, biomedicine and the world's traditional healing practices. A future *integrative paradigm* will incorporate understandings from genetics, the neurosciences, consciousness research, complexity theory and quantum field theory in addition to the evidence for the role of human intention in healing that is now emerging from studies.[26]

He cites a review of 23 controlled trials of different healing approaches which found that beneficial outcomes were reported in almost 60 per cent of cases where distant healing intention was used to treat medical or psychiatric disorders.

In the Brazilian integrative psychiatric hospitals, medical intuitives work as a team with a group of patients. They see the locus of the mind and spirit as being in the subtle body which is thought to envelop the physical body. It is here, at this subtle energetic level, that they believe healing can be brought about. Spiritual healing can be offered through hands-on energy passes or as distant healing intention, as mentioned by Lake in the controlled trials research.

Working with soul

The following case study illustrates how this kind of healing at the subtle energetic level can be applied in a Western consulting room. It helps bring it into a more familiar context for us. The case study is taken from an informative and moving chapter by British psychiatrist and psychotherapist Dr Andrew Powell in Emma Bragdon's edited collection.

Dr Powell has held consultant and academic positions in London and Oxford, including as Honorary Senior Lecturer in Psychotherapy at Oxford University. He is Founding Chair of the Special Interest Group on Spirituality and Psychiatry within the Royal College of Psychiatrists, and co-editor of *Spirituality and Psychiatry*. He has written several papers on spirituality and mental health in which he explores the possibilities of extending our understanding of scientific research and knowledge to include the spiritual dimension.

> A young woman came to see Dr Powell feeling not well and 'not herself'. She had been diagnosed as being clinically depressed. He particularly noticed her use of the phrase 'not myself'. It transpired that some months before the symptoms started, a friend had killed herself in the young woman's house. She had been staying there while Dr Powell's patient was away on holiday. By the time his patient returned, her friend's funeral was already over.[27]
>
> When asked, the young woman, who had held back for fear Dr Powell would think her mad, told him that 'every time she went into the house, she had the physical sensation that her friend was right there in the room with her'. Dr Powell asked if she would like him to invite the spirit of her deceased friend to the consultation. A conversation then took place, through the young woman, and Powell was able to help the deceased spirit move on towards the Light. The moment the spirit left, the young woman 'felt the burden of oppression lift from her and it did not return'.

This case study highlights a particular kind of psychospiritual therapeutic work, allowing deep healing to take place. Such soul-centred therapy is perhaps becoming culturally increasingly more accessible and acceptable today.

In answer to the question 'What is required when working with soul?' this is Dr Powell's valuable advice:

> First, a willingness to consider spiritual reality to be as 'real' as any aspect of life; second, a readiness to work beyond the bounds of consensus reality; and third, to trust that our patients already hold the key to their own healing, if only helped to make use of it.

Ancestral wounding

Another potential cause of our mental health struggles from the ancient indigenous perspective is where there is damaged ancestral energy which needs to be healed. Healing may be particularly helpful where we have taken on painful family patterns or where we may be carrying the results of intergenerational trauma, perhaps as the result of war or natural disaster. The original source is coming to the fore, ready to be tended to by a particular family member, sometimes after many, many generations. Something like a suicide, for instance, especially if it has been hushed up or become a family taboo, may impact on a person generations later. One effective way of healing this kind of ancestral wounding is through family constellations, which we covered under 'Healing approaches' on page 94. Significantly, as we saw, Bert Hellinger, the founder of the family constellations approach, lived in Africa for many years; his work was influenced by all he learnt there.

If you seek out healing from practitioners or transpersonal psychiatrists like Dr Andrew Powell who draw on the kind of wisdom we've covered in this chapter, it can be part of an integrative approach, alongside mainstream services. Take care, however, and be sure to follow the protocols we covered in Step 3 for checking their professional credentials. And trust your intuition. If something doesn't feel right, walk away.

Our mental health struggles have a meaning

We've seen that we have much to learn from the transpersonal wisdom of world traditions. The work of individuals such as Phil Borges, with his film *CrazyWise*, is now helping to bring this understanding more into the mainstream, to a wider audience. Even as

I write an exciting trend across Europe and America is emerging, becoming visible – a move to really bridge transpersonal and mainstream approaches to mental health. It is no coincidence that Sheldon Press invited me to write this book at this time. It is part of this emerging trend. There is a coming together of all those who want to see more holistic, more integrative, more humane mental health care, all those who believe that a mental health crisis holds the potential for healing and growth when properly understood, validated and supported: a coming together to speak with one voice, one strong voice. If you would like to find out about the emerging movement and add your voice to it you can find details on the 'Revisioning mental health' page of my website.

The integrative health movement is growing because it meets the needs of more and more people. More and more of us are realizing that our mental health struggles have a meaning. We are here to heal. People need to know that.

Finding the deeper meaning of our mental health struggles involves unearthing the causes of our distress. Sometimes there is not one single cause, but several; it is more a question of peeling away the layers. Sadly, old school psychiatry has in the past not been able or willing to explore such avenues. Through its reductionist biochemical model, it created a medical cul-de-sac. Fortunately, more and more of us are choosing not to go down it.

The transpersonal approach offers a much broader vista. We can begin to see our struggles from a new, bigger and bolder perspective. If we keep an open mind, we find a deeper meaning to our painful experiences. In time, as these act as a catalyst for our learning and growing, we come to be grateful for all that we've been through. We come to see our crisis for what it is, a gift.

End word

This book represents my vision for mental health, a vision where practitioners, including psychiatrists, are healers, where they are valued for the fantastic healing work they do. They have realized that prescribing psychiatric medication and simply controlling symptoms is not good enough, is not the answer. They have embraced change and trained in therapeutic methods that allow them to hear their patients and help them to heal. Above all, they know that growth and healing are possible for their patients. They validate their experiences and explain their symptoms to them, not in terms of illness but in terms of what is happening at the deeper level of soul and psyche. These practitioners and psychiatrists are not fearful. They have explored and embraced their own psyches, their own souls.

Already this vision is becoming a reality. Already the crisis within the field of mental health is proving to be a driver for change and evolution. But there is more. Mental health is not the only area in crisis. Today, we are being called as never before to respond to the global crisis we are facing across every sector of society. We are being called as never before to wake up, to wake up to a new level of consciousness, a higher level of consciousness, a level of consciousness which can respond creatively to our global crisis.

My book is based on the premise that a mental health crisis is an opportunity to do just that, to wake up to our true self. A quarter of the adult population in countries like the UK and the USA experiences some sort of mental health challenge in any one year, according to the Mental Health Foundation. Globally, the World Health Organization estimates that about 450 million people are struggling with their mental health. That's the number of people who are waking up . . . or who have the potential to do so.

When I see these numbers so starkly, I see something else *so* clearly. I see that the field of mental health holds the key to our collective awakening, the key to our transformation of consciousness. When we wake up in sufficient numbers we will reach a tipping point; we will collectively reach that higher level of consciousness from which to respond to the global crisis. As Einstein said,

'You can't solve a problem from the same level of consciousness as created it.'

Sometimes, when we look at the state of the world it can seem overwhelming. What can we as individuals do? If you are taking ownership of your journey towards healing, if you are seeking treatment that honours the deeper healing needs of your psyche and soul, if you are refusing to settle for anything less, know that you are making a difference. You are contributing to the healing of the Whole, to the awakening of the Whole.

Useful addresses

Organizations

Association for Transpersonal Psychiatry (Netherlands)
Website: www.transpsy.nl

Breathworks
Website: www.breathworks-mindfulness.org.uk

British Association for Counselling and Psychotherapy (BACP)
Website: www.bacp.co.uk

Center for Mindfulness in Medicine, Health Care, and Society, University of Massachusetts
www.umassmed.edu/cfm/

Centre for Counselling and Psychotherapy Education
Website: www.ccpe.org.uk

Centre for Mindfulness Research and Practice, Bangor University
Website: www.bangor.ac.uk/mindfulness/

Dances of Universal Peace
Website: www.dancesofuniversalpeace.org.uk

Depression Alliance
Website: www.depressionalliance.org

The Forgiveness Project
Website: http://theforgivenessproject.com

Hearing Voices Network
Website: www.hearing-voices.org
Resources on spirituality and hearing voices.

Hearing Voices Network USA
Website: www.hearingvoicesusa.org

Hearing Voices Network Wales
Website: http://hearingvoicescymru.org

Homeopathy Research Institute
Website: www.hri-research.org

Intervoice: The International Hearing Voices Network
Website: www.intervoiceonline.org

Karuna Institute: International Training and Retreat Centre
Website: www.karuna-institute.co.uk

London College of Psychic Studies
Website: www.collegeofpsychicstudies.co.uk

Mad in America
Website: www.madinamerica.com

Mind
Infoline: 0300 123 3393 or text 86463
Website: www.mind.org.uk

Refuge
24-hour National Domestic Violence Helpline: Freephone 0808 2000 247
Website: www.refuge.org.uk

Rethink
Website: www.rethink.org

Re-Vision: Centre for Integrative Psychosynthesis
Website: www.re-vision.org.uk

Royal College of Psychiatrists Spirituality and Psychiatry Special Interest Group
www.rcpsych.ac.uk/workinpsychiatry/specialinterestgroups/spirituality.aspx

Sane
Website: www.sane.org.uk
Includes an online support forum.

Self-injury Support
Website: www.selfinjurysupport.org.uk

Shiatsu Society
Website: www.shiatsusociety.org

Soteria Network
Website: www.soterianetwork.org.uk

Spiritual Crisis Network
Website: http://spiritualcrisisnetwork.uk

Spiritual Emergence Network (USA)
Website: http://spiritualemergence.info

Spiritual Emergence Network (Australia)
Website: www.spiritualemergence.org.au

Spiritual Emergence Service (SES) (Canada)
Tel.: (604) 533 3545
Free helpline: (604) 917 0117
Website: www.spiritualemergence.net

UK Council for Psychotherapy (UKCP)
Website: www.ukcp.org.uk

Windhorse Integrative Mental Health
Website: www.windhorseimh.org

Other resources

Directories

Counselling Directory
Website: www.counselling-directory.org.uk

Find a Homeopath
Website: www.findahomeopath.org.uk
Combines many of the different homeopath registers.

Films

CrazyWise, film directed by Phil Borges, see <www.crazywisefilm.com>.
'Spiritual emergency', episode of *Waking Universe*, featuring Catherine G.
    Lucas's interview with Lance Mungia, available on YouTube.
Take These Broken Wings, film by Daniel Mackler, available on YouTube.

Further information

Emma Bragdon
Website: http://emmabragdon.com

Kirtan and devotional chanting events
Website: www.naturalmysticbhajans.co.uk

Catherine G. Lucas
Website: www.catherine-g-lucas.com
Includes details of training.

Positive News
Website: http://positivenews.org.uk

References

1   Dr P. Bracken et al., 'Psychiatry beyond the current paradigm', *British Journal of Psychiatry*, 2012 (Dec.), 201(6), pp. 430–4.
2   A. Powell and C. MacKenna, 'Psychotherapy' in C. Cook, A. Powell and A. Sims (eds), *Spirituality and Psychiatry*, RCPsych Publications, London, 2009, p. 109.
3   R. Shorto, *Saints and Madmen*. Henry Holt, New York, 1999, p. 38.
4   Shorto, *Saints and Madmen*, p. 15.
5   Shorto, *Saints and Madmen*, p. 58.
6   John Weir Perry, *Trials of the Visionary Mind*. State University of New York Press, Albany, 1999, p. 23.
7   Perry, *Trials of the Visionary Mind*, p. 160.
8   Perry, *Trials of the Visionary Mind*, p. 164.
9   Michael O'Callaghan, 'A conversation with Dr John Weir Perry', <www.global-vision.org/papers/JWP.pdf>.
10 Perry, *Trials of the Visionary Mind*, p. 129.
11 Dr A. Powell, 'Soul-centered psychotherapy' in E. Bragdon (ed.), *Spiritism and Mental Health*, Singing Dragon, London, 2012, p. 181.
12 C. Myss, *Why People Don't Heal and How They Can*, Bantam Books, London, 1998, pp. 137–9.
13 In M. Aslan (ed.), *From Recovery to Emancipation: Stories of hope*. Crazy Diamond Publishing, Newton-le-Willows, 2008, pp. 19–21.
14 K. Mottram, *Mend the Gap*, Rethink Press, Great Britain, 2014, p. 117.
15 Mottram, *Mend the Gap*, p. 227.
16 J. Seikkula et al., 'Five years experiences of first-episode non affective psychosis in open dialogue approach: treatment principles, follow-up outcomes and two case studies', *Psychotherapy Research*, 16(2), pp. 214–28.
17 C. Scrivener, paper presented at the European Shiatsu Congress, October 2004.
18 K. Hall, 'Shiatsu in psychiatric care', *Shiatsu Society News*, 2010, 114 (Summer).
19 Reported by K. Hall in 'The treatment of mental-emotional conditions with Chinese medicine', *Shiatsu Society News*, 2004, 89 (Spring).
20 P. Adams, *Homeopathy: Good science*, Rhyme and Reason Books, Stroud, 2010, p. 52.
21 Adams, *Homeopathy: Good science*, p. 169.
22 J. Glenmullen, *Prozac Backlash*, Touchstone/Simon & Schuster, New York, 2000, p. 193.
23 R. Whitaker, *Anatomy of an Epidemic*, Broadway Paperbacks, New York, 2010, p. 110.
24 L. R. Mosher, 'Soteria and other alternatives to acute psychiatric hos-

pitalization: a personal and professional review', *Journal of Nervous and Mental Disease*, 1999, 187, pp. 142–9.

25 S. Marohn, *The Natural Medicine Guide to Bipolar Disorder*, Hampton Roads Publishing, Charlottesville, 2011, p. 173.

26 E. Bragdon (ed.), *Spiritism and Mental Health*, Singing Dragon, London 2012, p 5.

27 Powell, 'Soul-centered psychotherapy', pp. 184–5.

Further reading

Adams, P., *Homeopathy: Good science – how new science validates homeopathy*. Rhyme and Reason Books, Stroud, 2010.

Aron, E.N., *The Highly Sensitive Person: How to thrive when the world overwhelms you*. Element, London, 2003.

Aslan, M. (ed.) *From Recovery to Emancipation: Stories of hope*. Crazy Diamond Publishing, Newton-le-Willows, 2008, pp. 19–21.

Assagioli, R., *Psychosynthesis*. The Synthesis Center, Amherst, Massachusetts, 2000.

Assagioli, R., 'Self-realization and psychological disturbances', in S. and C. Grof (eds), *Spiritual Emergency: When personal transformation becomes a crisis*. Penguin Putnam, New York, 1990.

Bora, R. *Empowering People: Coaching for mental health recovery*, Rethink Mental Illness, London, 2012.

Bornhoft, G. and P. Matthiessen, *Homeopathy in Healthcare: Effectiveness, appropriateness, safety, costs*. Springer, Berlin, 2011.

Bracken, Dr P. et al, 'Psychiatry beyond the current paradigm', *British Journal of Psychiatry*, 2012 (Dec.), 201(6), pp. 430–4.

Bragdon, E. (ed.), *Spiritism and Mental Health*, Singing Dragon, London, 2012.

Breggin, Dr P., *Psychiatric Drug Withdrawal: A guide for prescribers, therapists, patients and their families*, Springer, New York, 2013.

Cameron, J., *The Artist's Way: A spiritual path to higher creativity*. Pan Books, London, 1995.

Cook, C., Powell, A. and Sims, A., *Spirituality and Psychiatry*. RCPsych Publications, London, 2009.

Dorman, Dr D., *Dante's Cure*. Other Press, New York, 2003.

Emoto, M., 'Healing with water', *Journal of Alternative and Complementary Medicine*, 2004, 10(1), pp. 19–21.

Emoto, M., *Hidden Messages in Water*. Atria Books, New York, 2005.

Fleischman, P., *The Healing Spirit: Explorations in religion and psychotherapy*. Paragon House, New York, 1989.

Frankl, V., *Man's Search for Meaning*. Rider, London, 2004 (originally published in German in 1946).

Ganio, M.S. et al., 'Human and clinical nutrition, mild dehydration impairs cognitive performance and mood of men', *British Journal of Nutrition*, 2011 (November), 106(10), pp. 1535–43.

Gilbert, P., *The Compassionate Mind (Compassion Focused Therapy)*. Constable, London, 2013.

Glenmullen, J., *Prozac Backlash*. Touchstone/Simon & Schuster, New York, 2000.

Grof, S. and C. (eds), *Spiritual Emergency: When personal transformation becomes a crisis*. Penguin Putnam, New York, 1989.

Grof, S. and C., *The Stormy Search for the Self*. Penguin Putnam, New York, 1990.

Hall, K., 'Shiatsu in psychiatric care', *Shiatsu Society News*, 2004 (Spring), p. 89.

Harrold, F. *Be Your Own Life Coach*. Hodder and Stoughton, London, 2000, pp. 109–14.

James, W., *The Varieties of Religious Experience*. Penguin, New York, 1982 (first published 1902).

Jamison, K.R., *An Unquiet Mind: A memoir of moods and madness*. Borzoi Books, New York, 1995.

Karon, Dr B., *Psychotherapy of Schizophrenia: The treatment of choice*. Rowman & Littlefield, Lanham, Maryland, 2004.

Kharitidi, O. *Entering the Circle: The secrets of ancient Siberian wisdom discovered by a Russian psychiatrist*. HarperCollins, New York, 1996.

Kingston, K., *Clear Your Clutter with Feng Shui*. Piatkus, London, 1998.

Laing, R.D., *The Politics of Experience*. Random House, London, 1967.

Laing, R.D. and Esterson, A., *Sanity, Madness and the Family*. Penguin, London, 1970 (first published 1964).

Lajoie, D.H. and Shapiro, S.I., 'Definitions of transpersonal psychology: the first twenty-three years', *Journal of Transpersonal Psychology*, 1992, 24(1), pp. 79–98.

Lake, J.H. and Spiegal, D. (eds), *Complementary and Alternative Treatments in Mental Health Care*. American Psychiatric Press, Arlington, Texas, 2006.

Linn, D., *Signposts: How to interpret the coincidences and symbols in your life*. Rider, London, 1996.

Lucas, C.G., *In Case of Spiritual Emergency*. Findhorn Press, Forres, 2011.

Lucas, C., *The Rainbow Journal*. Self-injury Support, Bristol, 2003.

Marohn, S., *The Natural Medicine Guide to Bipolar Disorder*. Hampton Roads Publishing, Charlottesville, Virginia, 2011.

May, Dr G.G., *The Dark Night of the Soul: A psychiatrist explores the connection between darkness and spiritual growth*. HarperOne, New York, 2005.

Mohr, T., *Playing Big: Find your voice, your vision and make things happen*. Hutchinson, London, 2014.

Mottram, K., *Mend the Gap: My transformative journey from deep despair to spiritual awakening*. Rethink Press, Gorleston, 2014.

Myss, C., *Why People Don't Heal and How They Can*. Bantam Books, London, 1998, pp. 137–9.

Perry, J.W., *The Far Side of Madness*. Spring Publications, Putnam, 2005.

Perry, J.W., *Trials of the Visionary Mind*. State University of New York Press, Albany, 1999.

Powell, Dr A., 'Soul-centered psychotherapy', in E. Bragdon (ed.), *Spiritism and Mental Health*, Singing Dragon, London, 2012.

Razzaque, Dr R., *Breaking Down is Waking Up*. Watkins Publishing, London, 2014.

Shorto, R., *Saints and Madmen*. Henry Holt, New York, 1999.

Somé, M.P., *Of Water and the Spirit*. Arkana, New York, 1995.

Sorrell, S., *Depression as a Spiritual Journey*. O Books, Winchester, 2009.

St Teresa of Ávila, *The Life of St Teresa of Ávila by Herself* (trans. J.M. Cohen). Penguin Books, London, 1957.

Wallcraft, Dr J., *Healing Minds: A report on current research policy and practice concerning the use of complementary and alternative therapies for a wide range of mental health problems*. London: Mental Health Foundation, 1998, Appendix 1: 'Choosing a practitioner of complementary therapies'.

Weil, Dr A., *Spontaneous Healing*. Warner Books, London, 1997.

Whitaker, R., *Anatomy of an Epidemic: Magic bullets, psychiatric drugs, and the astonishing rise of mental illness in America*. Broadway Paperbacks, New York, 2010.

Williams, M., Teasdale, J., Segal, Z. and Kabat-Zinn, J., *The Mindful Way through Depression*. The Guilford Press, New York, 2007.

Index